NCCN Guidelines for Patients®

The essential guide for people facing cancer.

Based on care recommendations from leading cancer experts.

Explains high-quality cancer care provided at state-of-the-art cancer centers.

Reviewed and revised every year.

Did you know that top cancer centers across the United States work together to improve cancer care? This alliance of leading cancer centers is called the National Comprehensive Cancer Network® (NCCN®).

Because cancer care is always evolving, NCCN develops and frequently updates evidence-based cancer care recommendations used by health care providers worldwide. These recommendations are known as the NCCN Clinical Practice Guidelines in Oncology (NCCN Guidelines®).

The NCCN Guidelines for Patients plainly explain these expert recommendations, so you can talk with your care team about the best care for you.

These NCCN Guidelines for Patients are based on the NCCN Guidelines® for Breast Cancer, Version 2.2026 — February 27, 2026.

View the NCCN Guidelines for Patients free online: NCCN.org/patientguidelines

Find an NCCN Cancer Center near you: NCCN.org/cancercenters

Learn how the NCCN Guidelines for Patients are developed: NCCN.org/patient-guidelines-process

Connect with us

@NCCNorg @NCCNVideo NCCN @NCCNorg

AF883711

Supporters

NCCN Guidelines for Patients are supported by funding from the NCCN Foundation®

NCCN Foundation gratefully acknowledges the following corporate supporters for helping to make available these NCCN Guidelines for Patients: AstraZeneca; Daiichi Sankyo; Genentech, Inc.; and Novartis Pharmaceuticals Corporation.

NCCN independently adapts, updates, and hosts the NCCN Guidelines for Patients. Our corporate supporters do not participate in the development of the NCCN Guidelines for Patients and are not responsible for the content and recommendations contained therein.

To make a gift, visit
NCCNFoundation.org/Donate

To learn more, visit online
NCCN.org/patientguidelines
or email
PatientGuidelines@NCCN.org

Contents

©2026 National Comprehensive Cancer Network, Inc. All rights reserved.

NCCN Guidelines for Patients and illustrations herein may not be reproduced in any form for any purpose without the express written permission of NCCN. No one, including doctors or patients, may use the NCCN Guidelines for Patients for any commercial purpose and may not claim, represent, or imply that the NCCN Guidelines for Patients that have been modified in any manner are derived from, based on, related to, or arise out of the NCCN Guidelines for Patients. The NCCN Guidelines are a work in progress that may be redefined as often as new significant data become available. NCCN makes no warranties of any kind whatsoever regarding its content, use, or application and disclaims any responsibility for its application or use in any way.

NCCN Foundation seeks to support the millions of patients and their families affected by a cancer diagnosis by funding and distributing NCCN Guidelines for Patients. NCCN Foundation is also committed to advancing cancer treatment by funding the nation's promising doctors at the center of innovation in cancer research. For more details and the full library of patient and caregiver resources, visit NCCN.org/patients.

National Comprehensive Cancer Network (NCCN) and NCCN Foundation
3025 Chemical Road, Suite 100, Plymouth Meeting, PA 19462 USA

1

About inflammatory breast cancer

In inflammatory breast cancer (IBC), cancer cells block lymph vessels in the skin of the breast. This causes the breast to look red and swollen and feel warm to the touch. Often, there's no lump that can be felt during a breast exam or seen on a mammogram. Treatment is a combination of drug therapy, surgery, and radiation therapy, which is explained in this guide.

What is inflammatory breast cancer?

Inflammatory breast cancer (IBC) is a type of invasive breast cancer. Invasive breast cancer is breast cancer that has grown into the surrounding tissue, lymph nodes, or breast skin. What makes IBC different from other breast cancers is its tendency to invade the drainage channels (lymphatics) of the breast and overlying skin. This causes the breast to rapidly swell with backed-up fluid and turn red as if inflamed.

Possible signs of IBC:

- Peau d'orange (pitted or dimpled appearance of skin)
- Skin thickening
- Edema (swelling caused by excess fluid in body tissue)
- Erythema (reddening of the skin, usually in patches

Inflammatory breast cancer

In inflammatory breast cancer (IBC), cancer cells block lymph vessels in the skin of the breast. This causes the breast to look red and swollen and feel warm to the touch.

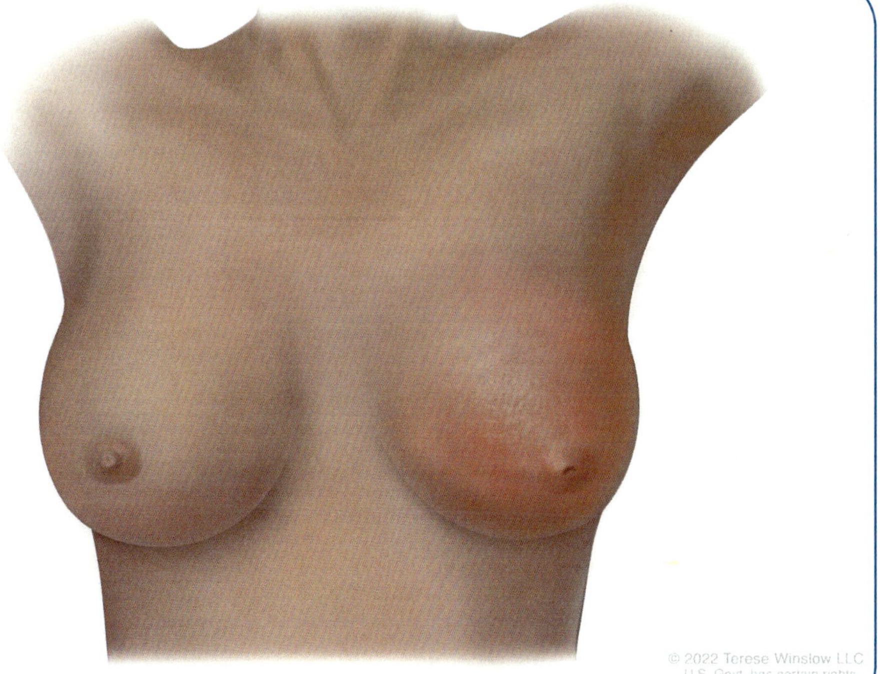

It's important not to dismiss any breast skin changes, including redness, swelling, or feeling warm to the touch. These changes could be an infection, but it's important to get medical attention right away.

What are the parts of the breast?

The breast is made of milk ducts, fat, nerves, lymph and blood vessels, ligaments, and other connective tissue. Behind the breast is the pectoral (chest) muscle and rib bones. Muscles and ligaments help hold the breast in place.

Breast tissue contains glands that can make milk. These milk glands are called lobules. Lobules look like tiny clusters of grapes. Small tubes called ducts connect the lobules to the nipple.

The ring of darker breast skin is called the areola. The raised tip within the areola is called the nipple. The nipple-areola complex is a term that refers to both parts.

Inflammatory breast cancer often starts in the ducts or lobules and spreads to surrounding breast tissue, lymph nodes, or skin. IBC can also spread to distant parts of the body.

How is inflammatory breast cancer treated?

Inflammatory breast cancer is treated with a combination of drug therapy, surgery, and radiation therapy. Treatment starts with drug therapy to shrink the tumor, followed by surgery to remove the breast and lymph nodes, and then radiation therapy to the chest wall and lymph nodes. Treatment aims to stop the spread of cancer.

Invasive ductal carcinoma

Most inflammatory breast cancers (IBCs) are invasive ductal carcinomas. This means that cancer started in the cells that line the milk ducts and has spread into surrounding tissue.

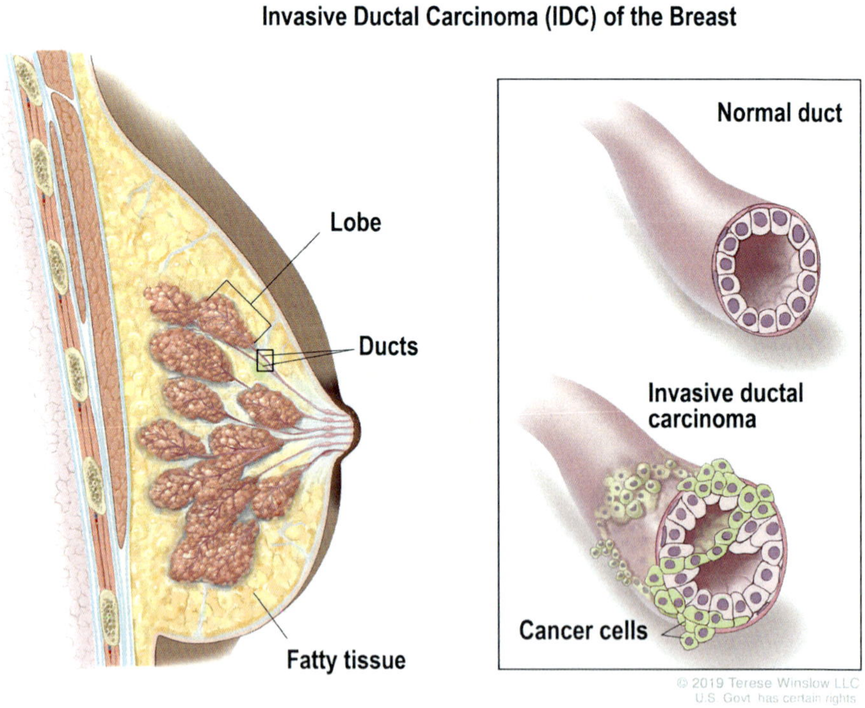

Like other breast cancers, IBC can develop in people assigned male at birth. Although there are some differences between breast cancers in people assigned male at birth and those assigned female, treatment is very similar for all genders.

How can I get the best care?

Advocate for yourself. You have an important role to play in your care. Many people feel more satisfied when they actively take part in planning their cancer care.

The NCCN Guidelines for Patients will help you play a larger role in your care. Discuss the recommendations in this guide with your care team. Ask questions about your options and share your goals and concerns.

Don't know what to ask? You're not alone. That's why we include suggested questions to ask at the end of chapters.

Keep reading to find the best care for you.

How this guide can help you

Making decisions about cancer care is stressful. There's a lot to learn, and you don't know what the future holds.

Use this guide to get the information and support you need.

Patients, doctors, and other health care professionals trust the NCCN Guidelines for Patients. This guide uses clear, everyday language to explain current cancer care recommendations made by respected experts in the field. Their recommendations are based on the latest research and practices at leading cancer centers.

Your health is unique to you, so your cancer care should be, too. As you read this guide, you'll learn which treatments are likely to provide the best results for you. And you'll be better prepared to talk with your care team.

"The NCCN Guidelines for Patients are seen as a trusted source by researchers, clinicians, and advocates. They set the standard for appropriate and effective breast cancer treatment, making them a good first step for newly diagnosed patients."

2

Testing for inflammatory breast cancer

Not all breast cancers are the same. Treatment planning starts with testing. This chapter presents an overview of the tests you might receive and what to expect.

Inflammatory breast cancer (IBC) can be difficult to diagnose. Often, there's no lump that can be felt during a breast exam or seen on a mammogram. Since there's swelling (edema) and redness (erythema) of the breast, IBC can look like an infection. A small skin biopsy of the affected breast area may help diagnose IBC. However, this doesn't replace a breast tissue biopsy. IBC is a clinical diagnosis, a biopsy-proven breast cancer with inflammatory features. You can have IBC even if a skin biopsy doesn't find breast cancer in the lymphatics of the skin.

Tests you might receive are listed in **Guide 1**.

General health tests

Medical history

A medical history is a record of all health issues and treatments you've had in your life. It asks about past surgeries and current health conditions. Bring a list of old and new medicines and any over-the-counter medicines, herbals, or supplements you take. Some supplements interact with and affect medicines that your care team may prescribe. Also tell your care team about any symptoms you have.

Family history

Some cancers and other diseases can run in families. Your care team will ask about the health history of family members who are blood relatives. This information is called family history. Ask members on both sides of your family about their health issues, like heart

Guide 1 Possible tests
Medical history and physical exam by a multidisciplinary team. Medical photographs will also be taken.
Biopsy with pathology review
Blood tests
Tumor estrogen receptor (ER) and progesterone receptor (PR) status
Tumor HER2 status
Fertility counseling for people not in menopause
Genetic counseling and testing if at risk of hereditary breast cancer
Distress screening
Imaging: • Diagnostic mammogram • Ultrasound and breast MRI, as needed • Chest CT. Contrast might be used. • CT or MRI of abdomen with or without pelvis. Contrast will be used. • Bone scan or FDG-PET/CT

disease, cancer, and diabetes, and at what age they were diagnosed. It's important to know their specific type of cancer, where the cancer started, if it's in multiple locations, and if they had genetic testing.

Physical exam

During a physical exam, your health care provider may:

- Check your temperature, blood pressure, pulse, and breathing rate
- Check your height and weight
- Listen to your lungs and heart
- Look in your eyes, ears, nose, and throat
- Feel and apply pressure to parts of your body to see if organs are of normal size, are soft or hard, or cause pain when touched.
- Examine your breasts to look for lumps, nipple discharge or bleeding, or skin changes.
- Feel for enlarged lymph nodes in your neck, armpit, and groin.

Clinical breast exam

Clinical breast exam is a physical exam of the bare breast performed by a health care provider to check for lumps or other changes. It's done while you're seated and/or lying down. Your provider should take time to palpate (feel) the entire breast, including the armpit. A nurse or assistant might also be in the room during the exam.

Your care team or doctor might ask to take pictures of the breast skin changes to document the areas involved before treatment is started. This information will help plan and guide surgery and radiation therapy.

Distress screening

Dealing with a cancer diagnosis can be stressful and may cause further distress. Distress is an unpleasant experience of a mental, physical, social, or spiritual nature. It can affect how you feel, think, and act. Distress might include feelings of sadness, fear, helplessness, worry, anger, and guilt. You may also have depression, anxiety, and sleep issues. Your treatment team will screen your level of distress. This is part of your cancer care.

Performance status

Performance status is a rating of a person's general level of fitness and ability to perform daily tasks. It includes whether you can walk, work, and take care of yourself. It's one factor taken into consideration when choosing a treatment plan.

Fertility (all genders)

Treatment with systemic therapy can affect your fertility, or the ability to have children. If you think you want children in the future, ask your care team how cancer treatment might affect your fertility.

Fertility preservation is all about keeping your options open, whether you know you want to have children later in life or aren't sure at the moment. Fertility and reproductive specialists can help you sort through what may be best for your situation.

More information on fertility preservation can be found in *NCCN Guidelines for Patients: Adolescent and Young Adult Cancer* NCCN.org/patientguidelines and on the NCCN Patient Guides for Cancer app.

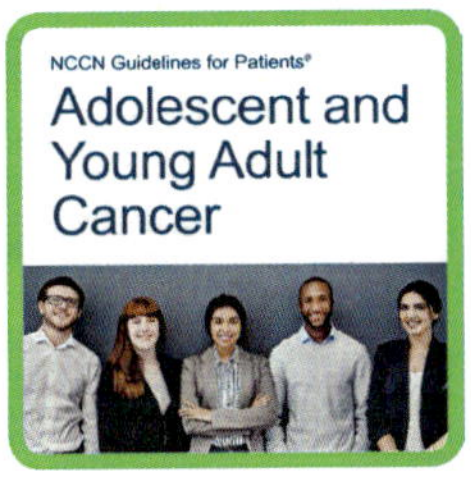

Preventing pregnancy during treatment

Preventing pregnancy during treatment is important. Cancer treatment can affect the ovaries, damage sperm, and hurt a developing baby. Therefore, becoming pregnant or having one's partner become pregnant during treatment should be avoided. If you are pregnant or breastfeeding at the time of your cancer diagnosis, treatments may need to be adjusted.

Blood tests

Blood tests check for signs of disease and how well organs are working. They require a sample of your blood, which is removed through a needle placed into a vein in your arm. Some blood tests you might have are described next.

Alkaline phosphatase level

Alkaline phosphatase (ALP) is an enzyme found in the blood. High levels of ALP can be a sign that cancer has spread to the bone or liver. A bone scan might be performed if you have high levels of ALP.

Inflammatory breast cancer can be difficult to diagnose. Ask for a referral to a breast specialist, if possible.

Complete blood count

A complete blood count measures the levels of red blood cells, white blood cells, and platelets in your blood. Red blood cells carry oxygen throughout your body, white blood cells fight infection, and platelets control bleeding.

Comprehensive metabolic panel

A comprehensive metabolic panel measures substances in your blood. It provides important information about how well your kidneys and liver are working, among other things.

Liver function tests

Liver function tests look at the health of your liver by measuring chemicals that are made or processed by the liver. Levels that are too high or low signal that the liver is not working well or that cancer has spread to the liver.

Pregnancy test

People who can become pregnant will be given a pregnancy test before treatment begins.

Imaging tests

Imaging tests take pictures of the inside of your body. These tests show where the cancer is located and the amount of the breast involved. A radiologist, a medical expert in interpreting imaging tests, will interpret the test and send a report to your care team.

Information about possible imaging tests are described next. They are listed in alphabetical order and not in order of importance.

Bone scan

The bone scan uses a radiotracer. A radiotracer is a substance that releases small amounts of radiation. Before the pictures are taken, the tracer is injected into your vein. It can take a few hours for the tracer to enter your bones.

A special camera takes pictures of the tracer in your bones. Areas of bone damage take up more radiotracer than healthy bone and show up as bright spots on the pictures. Bone damage can be caused by cancer, cancer treatment, previous injuries, or other health issues.

Bone x-ray

An x-ray uses low-dose radiation to take one picture at a time. A tumor changes the way radiation is absorbed and will show up on the x-ray. X-rays are also good at showing bone issues. Your care team may order x-rays if your bones hurt or were abnormal on a bone scan.

What's the difference between a screening and diagnostic mammogram?

A mammogram is a picture of the inside of your breast made using x-rays. During a mammogram, the breast is pressed between 2 plates while you stand in different positions. Multiple x-rays are taken. A computer combines the x-rays to make detailed pictures.

Screening mammogram

- Done on a regular basis when there are no signs or symptoms of breast cancer. Results take a few days.

Diagnostic mammogram

- Used for people with symptoms, such as a lump, pain, skin thickening or nipple discharge, or those whose breasts have changed shape or size. An ultrasound is often used with a diagnostic mammogram.
- Also used to take a closer look at an abnormal area found in a screening mammogram.
- A radiologist will evaluate the diagnostic mammogram while you wait so if additional testing is needed, it can be done right away.

Both types of mammograms use low-dose x-rays to examine the breast.

Contrast material

Contrast material is a substance used to improve the quality of imaging tests such as CT and MRI scans. It's used to make the pictures clearer. Not all imaging tests require contrast, but many do.

Contrast might be taken by mouth (oral) or given through a vein (intravenously or IV). The types of contrast vary and are different for CT and MRI.

Tell your care team if you've had allergic reactions to contrast in the past. This is important. You might be given medicines to avoid the effects of those allergies. Contrast might not be used if you have a serious allergy or if your kidneys aren't working well.

CT scan

A CT, or CAT, scan uses x-rays and computer technology to take pictures of the inside of the body. It takes many x-rays of the same body part from different angles. All of the images are combined to make one detailed picture. Contrast may or may not be used.

Diagnostic mammogram

A mammogram is a picture of the inside of your breast. The pictures are made using x-rays. A computer combines the x-rays to make detailed pictures. A bilateral mammogram includes pictures of both breasts. Mammogram results are used to plan treatment.

Diagnostic mammograms look at specific areas of your breasts, which may not be clearly seen on screening mammograms. Diagnostic mammograms include extra compression in certain areas of the breast, more magnification views, or rolling the breast to image additional areas. Other tests may include a breast MRI.

Breast MRI

If needed, a breast MRI will be done in addition to a mammogram. In a breast MRI, you're positioned face down with your arms overhead.

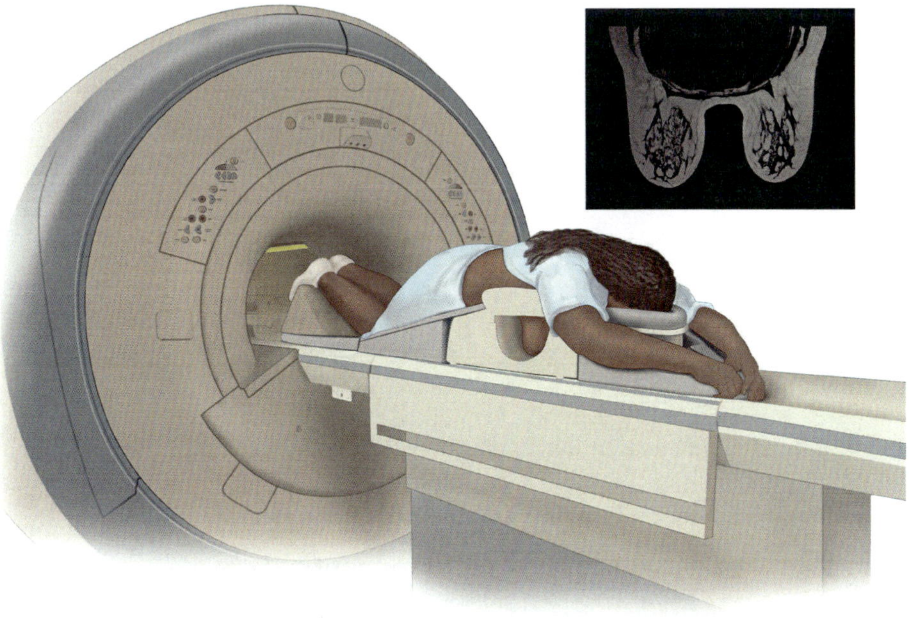

© 2022 Terese Winslow LLC
U.S. Govt. has certain rights

MRI scan

An MRI scan uses radio waves and powerful magnets to take pictures of the inside of the body. MRI doesn't use radiation. Because of the strong magnets used in the MRI machine, tell the technologist if you have any metal or a pacemaker in your body. Contrast is often used.

MRI scans take longer than CT scans. A closed MRI has a capsule-like design where the magnet surrounds you. The space is small and enclosed. An open MRI has a magnetic top and bottom, which allows for an opening on each end. Closed MRIs are more common than open MRIs, so if you have claustrophobia (a fear of enclosed spaces), be sure to tell your care team.

- **A breast MRI** might be used in addition to a mammogram. You will be positioned face down in the machine with your arms above your head. Sometimes, a breast MRI is used to guide a biopsy.
- **A spine or brain MRI** can be used to detect breast cancer that has spread (metastasized) to the spine or brain.

PET scan

A PET scan uses a radioactive substance called a tracer. A tracer is injected into a vein to see where the cancer cells are in the body and how much sugar they are taking up. This gives an idea about how fast the cancer cells are growing. Cancer cells show up as bright spots on PET scans. However, not all tumors appear on a PET scan. Also, not all bright spots found on the PET scan are cancer. It's normal for the brain, heart, kidneys, and bladder to be bright on a PET scan. Inflammation or infection can also show up as a bright spot.

When a PET scan is combined with CT, it's called a PET/CT scan. Types include:

- **FDG-PET/CT** uses a radiotracer called fluorodeoxyglucose (FDG). This scan is most helpful when other imaging results are unclear.
- **Sodium fluoride PET/CT** uses a radiotracer made of sodium fluoride.
- **FES-PET/CT** uses FES, which is a radioactive form of estrogen. An FES-PET/CT might be used when cancer is estrogen receptor-positive (ER+).

Ultrasound

An ultrasound uses high-energy sound waves to form pictures of the inside of the body. This is similar to the sonogram used for pregnancy. Gel will be applied to your bare breast, and a wand-like probe (transducer) will be held and moved around your breast and near your armpit. Ultrasound doesn't use x-rays, so it can be repeated as needed. Ultrasound is good at showing small areas of cancer that are near the skin. Sometimes, a breast ultrasound is used to guide a biopsy.

Biopsy

A biopsy removes a tissue sample from your body for testing. A pathologist will examine the biopsy for cancer and write a report called a pathology report.

There are different types of biopsies. Some biopsies are guided using imaging, such as ultrasound or MRI. The main tumor is biopsied first. Other tumors or tumors in different areas may also be biopsied. You may have tissue removed from the breast, lymph nodes, or both.

Types of possible biopsies include:

- **Fine-needle aspiration** and **core needle biopsy** use needles of different sizes to remove a sample of tissue or fluid.
- **Vacuum-assisted core biopsy** uses suction through a needle to remove the sample.
- **Excisional biopsy** removes the entire abnormal area. This isn't the preferred type of biopsy, but it may be necessary if other methods aren't possible or when the biopsy results don't match the expected findings. An excisional biopsy is usually done under anesthesia in an operating room.
- **Skin biopsy** takes a small sample of inflamed skin from the breast.

Before a biopsy, the area is usually injected with numbing medicine. A core needle biopsy removes more than one tissue sample, but usually through the same area on the breast. The samples are small. The needle is often guided into the tumor with imaging. When mammography is used during a biopsy, it's called a stereotactic needle biopsy.

Biopsy

In a biopsy, a sample of tumor is removed. There are different types of biopsy. This image shows an ultrasound-guided needle biopsy.

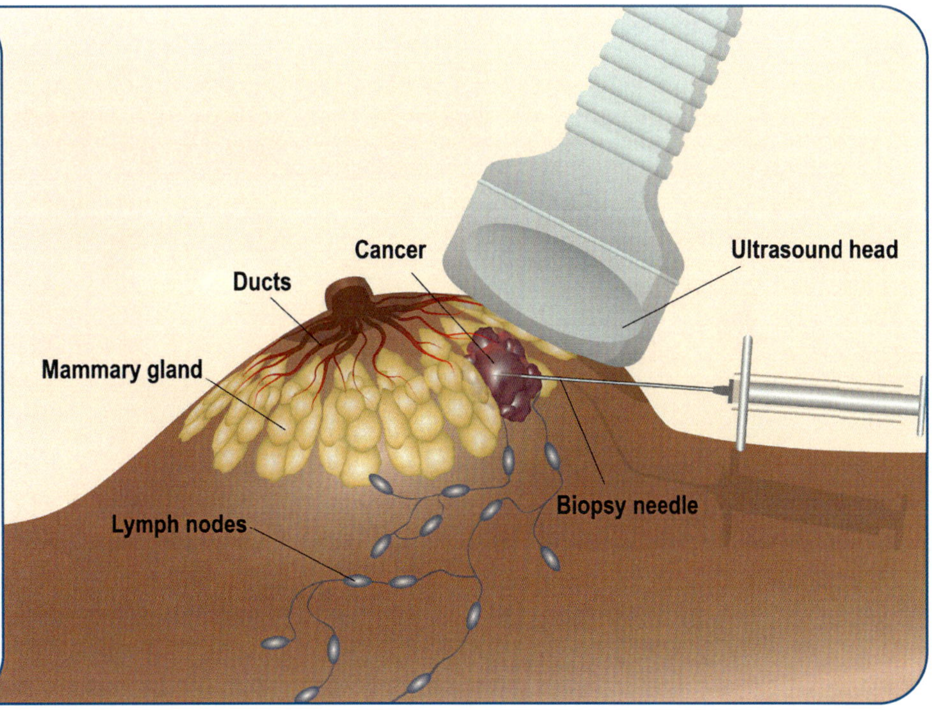

One or more clips may be placed near the breast tumor during a biopsy. The clips are small, painless, and made of metal. They mark the site for future treatment and imaging. The clips stay in place until surgery. If the area biopsied is benign, the clip will remain in place to mark the biopsy site in future imaging. The clips cause no problems, even if they're left in place for a long time. You'll be able to go through airport security and have an MRI.

Axillary lymph node needle biopsy

Axillary lymph nodes are found near the armpit. Axillary lymph nodes drain lymph fluid from the breast and nearby areas. In an axillary lymph node biopsy, a sample of lymph node near the armpit is biopsied with a needle. Since inflammatory breast cancer often affects the lymph nodes, this biopsy is used to determine if abnormal lymph nodes seen on imaging tests contain cancer cells. An ultrasound-guided fine-needle aspiration or core needle biopsy will be used. If cancer is found, it's called node positive (node+). A marker may be placed in the node so that it can be identified later during surgery.

Biopsy results

Your pathology report will contain information about histology. Histology is the study of the anatomy (structure) of cells, tissues, and organs under a microscope. It's used to make treatment decisions.

HER2 status

Inflammatory breast cancers often produce greater than normal amounts of human epidermal growth factor receptor 2 (HER2). HER2 is a protein involved in normal cell growth. It's found on the surface of all cells. When amounts are high, it causes cells to grow and divide. Some breast cancers have too many HER2 genes or receptors. This is called HER2-positive (HER2+) breast cancer. You might hear it called HER2 overexpression or amplification.

There are 2 tests for HER2:

- **Immunohistochemistry (IHC)** measures receptors. If the IHC score is 3+, the cancer is HER2+. If the score is 0 or 1, it's considered HER2-negative (HER2-). If the score is 2+, further testing is needed.
- **In situ hybridization (ISH)** counts the number of copies of the HER2 gene. This test is done mainly when the IHC score is unclear.

HER2 testing should be done on all new tumors or areas of concern. A biopsy sample will be used. You might have more than one HER2 test.

Immunohistochemistry

Immunohistochemistry (IHC) is a special staining process that involves adding a chemical marker to cancer or immune cells. The cells are then studied using a microscope. IHC can find estrogen, progesterone, and HER2 receptors in breast cancer cells. A pathologist will measure the number of cells with estrogen or progesterone receptors and the number of receptors inside each cell.

FISH or ISH

Fluorescence in situ hybridization (FISH), or other ISH methods like dual ISH, are testing methods that involve special dyes called probes that attach to pieces of DNA, the genetic material in a person's cells.

Hormone receptor status

Estrogen and progesterone are examples of hormones. A hormone is a substance made by a gland in your body. Hormones attach or bind to receptors found on the surface or inside certain cells.

When estrogen and progesterone attach to receptors found inside breast cancer cells, they can cause cancer to grow. Hormone receptor testing looks for estrogen and progesterone receptors in breast cancer cells. If found, these receptors may be targeted using endocrine (hormone-blocking) therapy.

Breast cancers can be hormone receptor-positive (HR+) or hormone receptor-negative (HR-). Hormone receptor testing should be done on any new tumors. A biopsy sample will be used.

Hormone receptor-positive

In hormone receptor-positive (HR+), or hormone-sensitive breast cancer, IHC finds estrogen receptors (ER+), progesterone hormone receptors (PR+), or both (ER+/PR+). Most breast cancers are ER+/PR+ or ER+/PR-. An ER-/PR+ tumor is relatively uncommon.

HR+ breast cancer can benefit from endocrine therapy, which blocks estrogen receptor signaling or decreases estrogen production.

Hormone receptor-negative

Hormone receptor-negative (HR-) breast cancer cells don't have estrogen or progesterone hormone receptors. These cancers are sometimes simply called hormone negative. HR- cancers often grow faster than HR+ cancers. Both the estrogen and progesterone receptors need to be negative for breast cancer to be considered HR-.

Biomarker testing

HER2 and hormone receptor status are part of biomarker testing. Your treatment team will recommend the best types of biomarker testing that are important for you.

Biomarker testing includes tests of genes or their products (proteins). It identifies the presence or absence of mutations and certain proteins that might suggest treatment. Proteins are written like this: BRCA. Genes are written with italics like this: *BRCA*.

Mutation testing is more commonly done in metastatic breast cancer. For more information, see *NCCN Guidelines for Patients: Metastatic Breast Cancer* at NCCN.org/patientguidelines and on the NCCN Patient Guides for Cancer app.

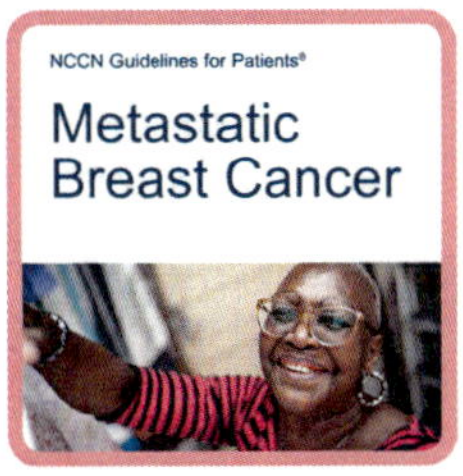

Tumor mutation testing

A sample of your tumor or blood may be used to see if the cancer cells have any specific DNA mutations. This testing differs from the genetic testing for mutations you may have inherited from your birth parents. In tumor mutation testing, only the tumor is tested.

Testing is done using a variety of methods such as FISH, ISH, IHC, next-generation sequencing (NGS), and/or polymerase chain reaction (PCR). These methods are used to identify the presence of gene mutations, alterations, rearrangements, or fusions found in the tumor. Currently, these findings are only useful for stage 4 breast cancer, but this could change.

- Certain mutations such as *PIK3CA, AKT1, PTEN, ESR1, NTRK*, and *RET* can be targeted with specific therapies.
- Testing for *ESR1* and *RET* mutations is done on hormone receptor-positive (HR+) tumors.

PD-L1 testing

Programmed death ligand 1 (PD-L1) is an immune protein. If this protein is expressed on the surface of cancer cells, it can cause your immune cells to ignore the cancer and suppress the anti-tumor immune response. If your cancer expresses PD-L1, you might have treatment that combines chemotherapy and an immune checkpoint inhibitor therapy. This is designed to activate your immune system to better fight off the cancer cells.

Testing takes time. It might take days or weeks before all test results come in.

Tumor mutational burden

When there are 10 or more mutations per million base pairs of tumor DNA, it's called tumor mutational burden-high (TMB-H). TMB-H can be used to help predict response to cancer treatment using immune checkpoint inhibitors that target the protein PD-L1.

MSI-H/dMMR mutation

Microsatellites are short, repeated strings of DNA. When errors or defects occur, they are fixed by mismatch repair (MMR) proteins. Some cancers have DNA mutations for changes that prevent these errors from being fixed. This is called microsatellite instability (MSI) or MMR deficient (dMMR). When cancer cells have more than a normal number of microsatellites, it's called MSI-high (MSI-H). This is often due to dMMR genes.

Tumor markers

Your blood or biopsy tissue may be tested for proteins called tumor markers. Knowing this information can help plan treatment. Examples of some tumor markers in breast cancer include carcinoembryonic antigen (CEA), CA 15-3, and CA 27.29. An increase in the level of certain tumor markers could mean the cancer has grown or spread (progressed). However, not everyone has elevated levels of these markers, and tumor markers alone are not a reliable method of detecting breast cancer.

Therefore, they aren't routinely checked and depend on your individual situation.

Liquid biopsy

Some abnormal changes (mutations) can be found by testing circulating tumor DNA (ctDNA) in the blood. In a liquid biopsy, a sample of blood is taken to look for cancer cells or for pieces of DNA from tumor cells. Sometimes, testing can quickly use up a tumor sample, and a liquid biopsy might be an option in this case.

Genetic cancer risk testing

About 1 out of 20 breast cancers are hereditary, which means they are passed down from birth parents through DNA. Depending on your family history or other features of your cancer, your health care provider might refer you for genetic counseling and hereditary genetic testing to learn more about your cancer. A genetic counselor or trained provider will speak with you about the results. Test results may guide treatment planning.

Genetic testing is done using blood or saliva. The goal is to look for gene mutations inherited from your biological (birth) parents, called germline mutations. Some mutations can put you at risk for more than 1 type of cancer. You can pass these genes on to your children. Also, other family members might carry these mutations. Tell your care team if there's a family history of cancer.

More information on genetic cancer risk testing can be found in *NCCN Guidelines for Patients: Genetic Testing for Hereditary Breast, Ovarian, Pancreatic, and Prostate Cancers* NCCN.org/patientguidelines and on the NCCN Patient Guides for Cancer app.

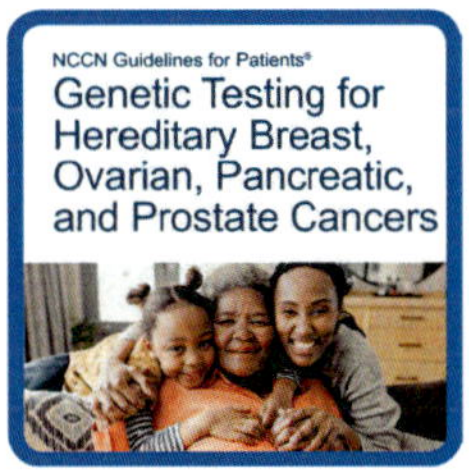

BRCA mutation tests

Everyone has *BRCA* genes. Normal *BRCA* genes help to prevent tumor growth, help fix damaged cells, and help cells grow normally. However, mutations in *BRCA1* or *BRCA2* increase the risk of breast, ovarian, prostate, colorectal, pancreatic, and melanoma skin cancers. Mutated *BRCA* genes can also affect how some treatments work.

The technology for genetic testing has improved, so if you tested negative for a gene mutation over 10 years ago, you may be re-tested.

Other genes that might be tested

Other genes, such as *PALB2, p53, CHEK2,* and *ATM*, might be tested. For example, *PALB2* normally helps prevent cancer. When *PALB2* mutates, it no longer works correctly. People with a *PALB2* mutation have a higher risk of developing breast cancer.

Key points

- Inflammatory breast cancer (IBC) can be difficult to diagnose. Often, there is no lump that can be felt during a breast exam or seen on a mammogram. Since IBC can look like an infection, a biopsy of the affected skin may help diagnose IBC. However, this doesn't replace a breast tissue biopsy.
- An axillary lymph node biopsy removes a sample of lymph node near the armpit. Since inflammatory breast cancer often affects the lymph nodes, an axillary lymph node biopsy may be needed.
- A sample from a biopsy of your tumor will be tested for estrogen receptor (ER) status, progesterone receptor (PR) status, HER2 status, and grade (histology). IBC can vary in its expression of these receptors and isn't confined to 1 subtype of breast cancer.
- Biomarker testing provides information about the behavior of your cancer, as well as treatments your cancer may respond to.
- Treatment can affect your fertility or the ability to have children. You might be referred to a fertility specialist to discuss fertility preservation.
- About 1 out of 20 breast cancers are hereditary. Depending on your family history or other features of your cancer, your health care provider might refer you for hereditary genetic testing or to a genetic counselor.

Questions to ask

- What type(s) of biopsy will I have? Will I have a skin biopsy?
- What tests will be done on the tumor?
- When will the test results be ready and who will discuss them with me?
- What is the tumor HER2 and hormone receptor status?
- What tumor features or mutations will you test for?

What's next?

The next chapter provides information on breast cancer staging. At diagnosis, most inflammatory breast cancers are stage 3 or 4.

"For weeks my bra had been feeling uncomfortably tight. I tried to ignore it but then felt sharp, shooting pains and the skin looked 'funny.' It took multiple office visits and finally to a surgeon to learn I had inflammatory breast cancer (IBC). I'm a nurse and didn't know you could have breast cancer without a lump."

3
Breast cancer staging

Cancer staging is used to guide treatment decisions. It describes the size and location of the tumor and if cancer has spread to lymph nodes, organs, or other parts of the body. It also considers hormone receptor (HR) and HER2 status, and standard-of-care treatment results.

Most inflammatory breast cancers (IBCs) are invasive ductal carcinomas. This is cancer that started in the cells that line the milk ducts and has spread into surrounding tissue. At diagnosis, IBC is stage 3 or 4 disease. In stage 3, the tumor can be any size and in the lymph nodes, the lymph nodes can be fixed (or not moveable), or the cancer can involve the skin or chest wall. It's sometimes called advanced disease. In stage 4, cancer has spread to other parts of the body (metastasized).

IBC is a clinical diagnosis, a biopsy-proven breast cancer with inflammatory features. That means an IBC diagnosis requires evidence of cancer from a biopsy along with breast and skin changes over a large portion of the breast (over one-third of the breast) that develop in a short period of time (less than 6 months). Sometime a diagnosis for IBC can be challenging to make, and some physicians will use a scoring system to assist in determining the likelihood you have IBC. These scoring systems, like the Inflammatory Breast Cancer (IBC) Scoring System from the Komen Foundation, can assist in a clinical diagnosis.

More information about breast cancer staging is explained next.

How is breast cancer staged?

A cancer stage is a way to describe the extent of the cancer at the time you are first diagnosed. Based on testing, your cancer will be assigned a stage. Staging helps to predict prognosis and is needed to make treatment decisions. A prognosis is the course your cancer will likely take.

Information gathered during staging:

- **The extent (size) of the tumor (T)**: How large is the cancer? Has it grown into nearby areas?
- **The spread to nearby lymph nodes (N)**: Has the cancer spread to nearby lymph nodes? If so, how many? Where?
- **The spread (metastasis) to distant sites (M)**: Has the cancer spread to distant organs such as the lungs or liver?
- **Hormone receptor (HR) status**: Does the cancer have estrogen receptors (ER) or progesterone receptors (PR)?
- **HER2 status**: Does the cancer make too much of a protein called HER2?
- **Grade of the cancer (G)**: How much do the cancer cells look like normal cells?
- **Biomarker testing**: Does the cancer have any genes, proteins, markers, or mutations that might suggest treatment?

Staging is based on a combination of information to reach a numbered stage. It takes into account what can be felt during a physical exam, what can be seen on imaging tests, and what is found during a biopsy or surgery. Often, not all information is available at the initial evaluation. More information can be gathered as treatment begins.

Staging includes:

- **Anatomic** – Based on the extent of cancer as defined by tumor size (T), lymph node status (N), and distant metastasis (M).
- **Prognostic** – Includes anatomic TNM plus tumor grade and the status of the biomarkers such as human epidermal growth factor receptor 2 (HER2), estrogen receptor (ER), and progesterone receptor (PR). Prognostic stage also includes the assumption that you are being treated with the standard-of-care approaches.

Breast cancer staging is often done twice, before and after surgery. Staging after surgery provides more specific and accurate details about the size of the cancer and lymph node status.

Clinical stage

Clinical stage (c) is the rating given before any treatment. An example might look like cT1 or cN2. In breast cancer, the clinical stage is based on imaging and biopsy results. These tests are done as part of an initial diagnosis before any treatment.

Pathologic stage

Pathologic stage (p) or surgical stage is determined by examining tissue removed during surgery. An example might be pN2. If you are given drug therapy before surgery, then the stage might add a y and look like ypT3.

Clinical staging

Clinical staging of lymph nodes is staging before surgery.

- **Cancer is in axillary nodes**
- **Cancer is in internal mammary nodes**
- **Cancer is in infraclavicular nodes**
- **Cancer is in supraclavicular nodes**

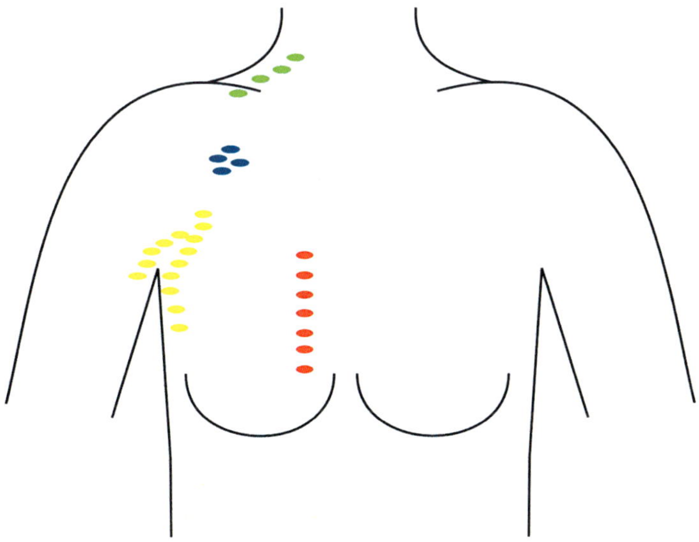

TNM scores

The tumor, node, and metastasis (TNM) system is used to stage breast cancer. In this system, the letters T, N, and M describe different areas of cancer growth. Based on cancer test results, your doctor will assign a score or number to each letter. The higher the number, the larger the tumor or the more the cancer has spread. These scores will be combined to assign the cancer a stage. A TNM example might look like this: T3N2M0 or T3, N2, M0.

T = Tumor

T describes the depth and size of the main tumor in 1 or both breasts. Tumor size can be measured in centimeters (cm) or millimeters (mm). One inch is equal to 2.54 cm. For comparison, a large pea is 1 cm (10 mm) and a 1 golf ball is 4 cm (40 mm). A tumor micrometastasis is a very small collection of cancerous cells smaller than 1 mm. It might be written as T1mi. Ipsilateral means on the same side of the body.

- **T1** – Tumor is 2 cm (20 mm) or less
- **T2** – Tumor is 2.1 cm to 5 cm
- **T3** – Tumor is more than 5 cm
- **T4** – Tumor is of any size and has invaded nearby structures such as the chest wall and skin of the breast
- **T4d** – Tumor is inflammatory carcinoma (inflammatory breast cancer)

N = Regional lymph node

Lymph, a clear fluid containing cells that help fight infections and other diseases, drains through channels into lymphatic vessels. From here, lymph drains into lymph nodes. Lymph nodes work as filters to help fight infection.

Regional lymph nodes are located near the breast in the armpit (axilla). If breast cancer spreads, it often goes first to nearby lymph nodes under the arm. It can also sometimes spread to lymph nodes near the collarbone or near the breastbone. However, it's possible for cancerous cells to travel through lymph and blood to other parts of the body without having gone to the lymph nodes first. Knowing if the cancer has spread to your lymph nodes helps doctors find the best way to treat your cancer.

- **N0** – No cancer is found in the regional lymph nodes. Isolated tumor cells may be present. These are malignant cell clusters no larger than 0.2 mm.
- **N1mi** – Micrometastases (approximately 200 cells, larger than 0.2 mm, but not larger than 2.0 mm) are found in lymph nodes.
- **N1, N2, N3** – Regional lymph node metastases are found. The higher the number, the more lymph nodes that have metastases.

M = Metastasis

Cancer can spread to distant parts of the body. The most common sites for metastasis are bone and lung.

- **M0** – No evidence of distant metastasis.
- **M1** – Distant metastasis is found. This is metastatic breast cancer.

Grade

Grade describes how abnormal tumor cells look under a microscope (called histology). Higher-grade cancers tend to grow and spread faster than lower-grade cancers. G3 is the highest grade for breast cancers. A low-grade tumor has a low risk of cancer returning (called recurrence). A high-grade tumor has a higher risk of recurrence.

- **GX** – Grade cannot be determined
- **G1** – Low
- **G2** – Intermediate
- **G3** – High

Breast cancer stages

Numbered stages are based on TNM scores and hormone receptor and HER2 status. Stages range from stage 0 to stage 4, with 4 being the most advanced. They might be written as stage 0, stage I, stage II, stage III, and stage IV. Inflammatory breast cancer (IBC) is stage 3 (invasive) or 4 (metastatic).

- **Stage 0 is noninvasive** – Noninvasive breast cancer is rated stage 0. It hasn't spread to the surrounding breast tissue, lymph nodes, or distant sites.
- **Stages 1, 2, and 3 are invasive but not metastatic** – Invasive breast cancer is rated stage 1, 2, or 3. It has grown outside of the ducts, lobules, or breast skin. Cancer might be in the axillary lymph nodes.
- **Stage 4 is metastatic** – In stage 4 breast cancer, cancer has spread to distant sites. It can develop from earlier stages. Sometimes, the first diagnosis is stage 4 metastatic breast cancer (called de novo).

Key points

- The tumor, node, and metastasis (TNM) system is used to stage breast cancer. Inflammatory breast cancer is either stage 3 or 4 at diagnosis and is a clinical diagnosis. This means there needs to be evidence of cancer along with breast and skin changes and other features.
- Scoring systems may be helpful in determining the likelihood you have inflammatory breast cancer.
- Breast cancer is often staged twice, before and after surgery.
- Clinical stage is the rating given before any treatment.
- Pathologic stage or surgical stage is determined by examining tissue removed during surgery.
- Grade describes how abnormal tumor cells look under a microscope (called histology).
- Regional lymph nodes are found near the breast.

Questions to ask

- What is the cancer stage and tumor grade?
- What is the likelihood I have inflammatory breast cancer based on the Inflammatory Breast Cancer (IBC) Scoring System?
- What does the cancer stage and grade mean in terms of treatment options and prognosis?
- Is cancer in the lymph nodes? If so, which lymph nodes?
- What is the tumor HER2 and hormone status?

What's next?

The next chapter provides information on the types of treatment and what to expect.

4

Types of treatment

This chapter provides an overview of treatment options and what to expect. Together, you and your care team will choose a treatment plan that's best for you.

Your care team

Treating cancer takes a team approach. Treatment decisions should involve a team of health care and psychosocial care professionals from different backgrounds who have knowledge and experience in your type of cancer. This team is united in planning and implementing your treatment.

Treatment overview

Inflammatory breast cancer (IBC) is treatable. It's treated with systemic (drug) therapy to shrink the tumor, followed by surgery to remove the breast and lymph nodes, and then radiation therapy. Surgery isn't always possible. Treatment is based on tumor estrogen receptor (ER), progesterone receptor (PR), and HER2 expression.

Many factors play a role in how your cancer will respond to treatment. It's important to have regular talks with your care team about your goals for treatment and your treatment plan.

The best-known way to treat a particular disease based on past clinical trials is called standard of care. There may be more than one treatment considered standard of care. Ask your care team what treatment options are available and if a clinical trial might be right for you.

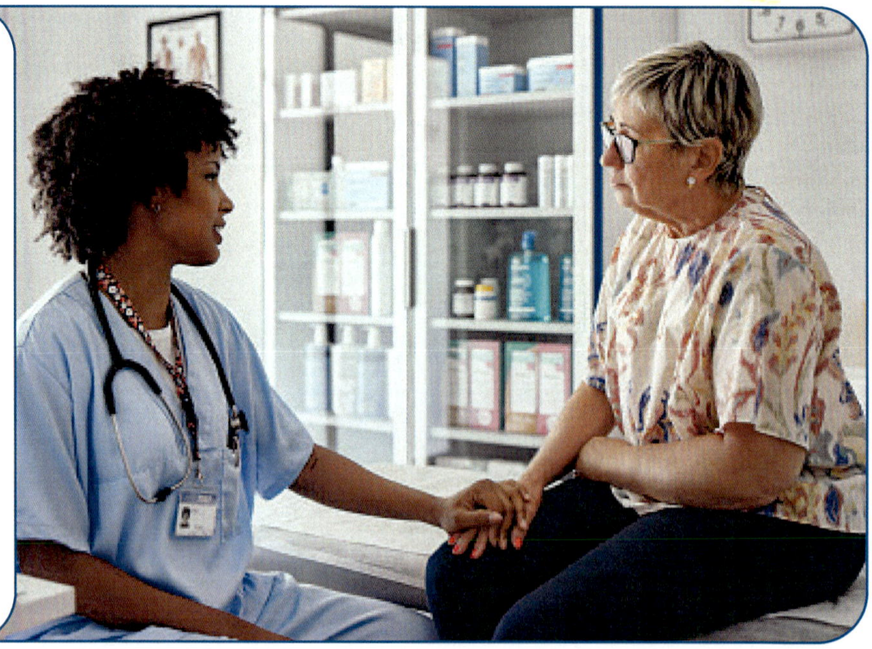

Mastectomy

Inflammatory breast cancer is often treated with a modified radical mastectomy. In a modified radical mastectomy, the breast and underarm (axilla) lymph nodes are removed.

When preparing for surgery, seek the opinion of an experienced surgeon. The surgeon should be an expert in your type of surgery. Hospitals that perform many surgeries often have better results. You can ask for a referral to a hospital or cancer center that has experience in treating your type of cancer.

Breast reconstruction is an option after a mastectomy. If you opt for reconstruction, it will be done after you finish cancer treatment. This is called delayed reconstruction. Breast reconstruction is often done in stages. You might want to consult with a plastic surgeon.

"When I was diagnosed with inflammatory breast cancer (IBC) the doctor told me to stay away from the Internet, but I wanted to learn all I could. You need to learn so you can advocate for yourself. Not everyone has experience treating this disease. Just be sure to go to reputable sources for information."

Modified radical mastectomy

In a modified radical mastectomy, the entire breast and some lymph nodes are removed (dotted line).

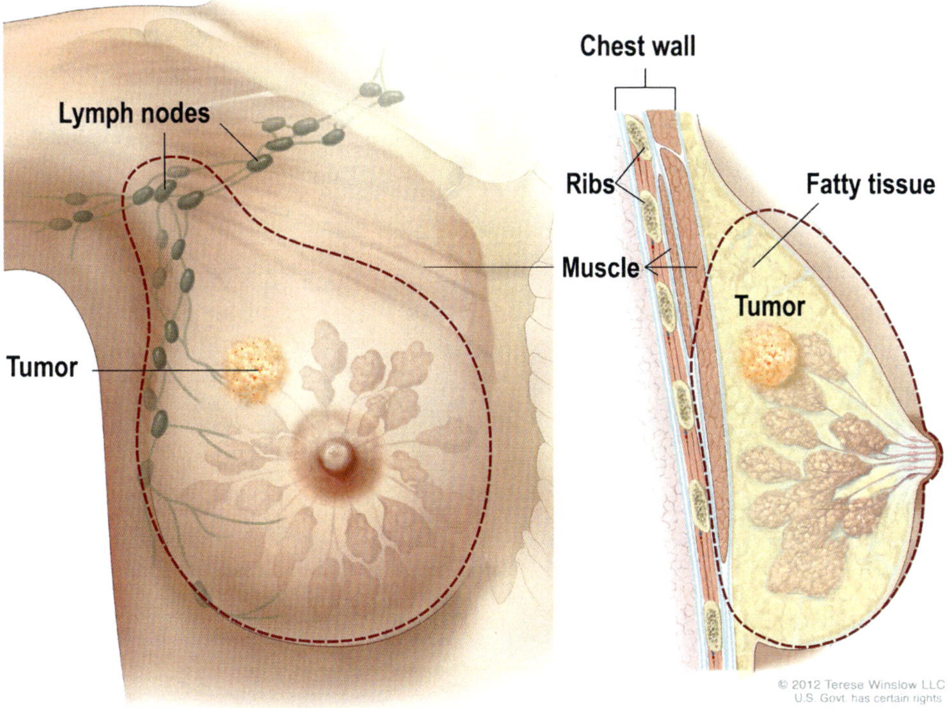

Axillary lymph node dissection

Axillary lymph node dissection (ALND) is done at the time of a mastectomy to remove lymph nodes found near the armpit. This is performed after an axillary lymph node biopsy shows cancer in the lymph nodes (called node positive). The ALND will remove any lymph nodes that contain cancer. Removing lymph nodes can cause lymphedema (fluid buildup) and other health issues.

When the axillary nodes are removed with the breast, it's called a modified radical mastectomy.

There are 3 levels of axillary lymph nodes:

- **Level I** – Nodes located below the lower edge of the chest muscle
- **Level II** – Nodes located underneath the chest muscle
- **Level III** – Nodes located above the chest muscle near the collarbone

An ALND usually removes level I and II axillary lymph nodes. For more information about the timing of biopsies, talk with your care team.

Axillary lymph node dissection

Axillary lymph node dissection (ALND) is done at the time of a mastectomy to remove lymph nodes found near the armpit. The ALND removes any lymph nodes with cancer.

Level I

Level II

Level III

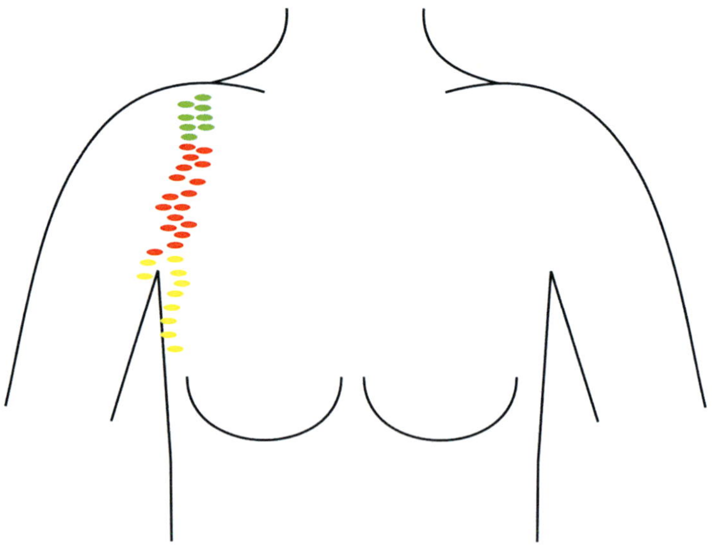

Radiation therapy

Radiation therapy (RT) uses high-energy radiation from x-rays (photons), protons, and other sources to kill any cancer cells that remain after a mastectomy. It's a standard part of inflammatory breast cancer treatment.

You will see your radiation oncologist at least weekly to discuss treatment results and to help with any side effects, such as a sunburn-like rash. Ask your care team which radiation option(s) are best for your situation, if radiation therapy will be combined with drug therapy, and what side effects to expect.

Systemic therapy

Systemic therapy is drug therapy that works throughout the body. It's one part of an inflammatory breast cancer treatment plan.

All systemic treatments listed in this guide are recommended and appropriate. When helpful, NCCN experts also assign a level of preference to their recommendations for systemic therapies:

- **Preferred therapies** have the most evidence they may work better and be safer than other therapies.
- **Other recommended therapies** can provide effective results but may have less evidence, more side effects, or may not work quite as well as preferred therapies.
- **Therapies used in certain cases** work best for individuals with specific cancer features or health circumstances.

For a general list of systemic therapies, see **Guide 2**.

Systemic therapies are described in more detail below and in the following pages.

Chemotherapy

Chemotherapy kills fast-dividing cells throughout the body, including cancer cells and some normal cells. More than 1 chemotherapy may be used to treat inflammatory breast cancer. When only 1 drug is used, it's called a single agent. A combination or multi-agent regimen is the use of 2 or more chemotherapy drugs.

Some chemotherapy drugs are liquids given through a vein or injected under the skin with a needle. Other chemotherapy drugs may be given as a pill that's swallowed.

Most chemotherapy is given in cycles of treatment days followed by days of rest. This allows the body to recover before the next cycle. Cycles vary in length depending on which drugs are used. The number of treatment days per cycle and the total number of cycles given also vary.

Antibody drug conjugates

An antibody drug conjugate (ADC) delivers cell-specific chemotherapy. It attaches to a protein found on the outside of the cancer cell, then enters the cell. Once inside the cell, chemotherapy is released. ADCs are given in cycles. Some ADCs target HER2.

Guide 2
Systemic therapy examples (listed in alphabetical order)

Chemotherapy	• Capecitabine (Xeloda) • Carboplatin (Kyxata) • Cisplatin • Cyclophosphamide (Frindovyx) • Docetaxel • Doxorubicin (Doxi) • Epirubicin (Ellence) • Eribulin (Halaven) • Fluorouracil • Gemcitabine (Avgemsi) • Methotrexate • Paclitaxel • Vinorelbine
Antibody drug conjugate (ADC)	• Ado-trastuzumab emtansine (T-DM1) (Kadcyla) • Datopotamab deruxtecan-dlnk (Datroway) • Fam-trastuzumab deruxtecan-nxki (T-DXd) (Enhertu) • Sacituzumab govitecan-hziy (Trodelvy)
Targeted therapy (these don't target HER2)	CDK4/6 inhibitors • Abemaciclib (Verzenio), Palbociclib (Ibrance), and Ribociclib (Kisqali)
	PARP inhibitors • Olaparib (Lynparza) and Talazoparib (Talzenna)
	PIK3CA, AKT1, PTEN, ROS1, TRK, mTOR, and other inhibitors • Alpelisib (Piqray), Capivasertib (Truqap), Entrectinib (Entrectinib), Erdafitinib (Balversa), Everolimus (Afinitor), Inavolisib (Itovebi), Larotrectinib (Vitrakvi), Repotrectinib (Augtyro), and Selpercatinib (Retevmo)
HER2-targeting therapy	Antibodies • Margetuximab-cmkb (Margenza) • Pertuzumab (Perjeta) and its substitutes called biosimilars • Trastuzumab (Herceptin) and biosimilars
	ADCs • Ado-trastuzumab emtansine and Fam-trastuzumab deruxtecan-nxki
	Inhibitors • Lapatinib (Tykerb), Neratinib (Nerlynx), and Tucatinib (Tukysa)
Immunotherapy	• Pembrolizumab (Keytruda) and Dostarlimab-gxly (Jemperli)
Endocrine therapy	• Endocrine therapy can be found in **Guide 3.**

HER2-targeted therapy

When breast cancer has higher amounts of HER2, it's called HER2-positive (HER2+) breast cancer.

HER2-targeted therapy treats HER2+ breast cancer. Some HER2-targeted therapy is given with chemotherapy. However, it might be used alone or in combination with endocrine therapy.

HER2-targeted therapies include:

- **HER2 antibodies** prevent HER2 growth signals from outside of the cell. They also help immune cells attack cancer cells.
- **HER2 inhibitors** stop HER2 growth signals from within the cell.
- **HER2 conjugates or HER2 antibody drug conjugates (ADCs)** deliver cell-specific chemotherapy. They attach directly to HER2s, then enter the cell. Once inside, chemotherapy is released.

Your heart will be monitored before and during treatment with HER2-targeted therapy. Tests will measure the left ventricular ejection fraction, the amount of blood pumping from the left side of the heart.

Other targeted therapies

This section discusses inhibitors that are different from inhibitors used in HER2-targeted therapy.

CDK4/6 inhibitors

CDK is a cell protein that helps cells grow and divide. For hormone receptor-positive (HR+) with HER2-negative (HER2-) cancer, taking a CDK4/6 inhibitor with endocrine therapy may help control cancer longer and improve survival. CDK4/6 inhibitors include abemaciclib, palbociclib, and ribociclib.

PARP inhibitors

Cancer cells often become damaged. PARP is a cell protein that repairs cancer cells and allows them to survive. Blocking PARP can cause cancer cells to die. Olaparib and talazoparib are examples of PARP inhibitors (PARPi).

PIK3CA, AKT1, PTEN, and other inhibitors

The *PIK3CA* gene is one of the most frequently mutated genes in breast cancers. The *PTEN* and *AKT* genes can also be altered in breast cancers. A mutation or alteration in any of these genes can lead to increased growth of cancer cells and resistance to various treatments. Alpelisib and inavolisib are examples of a PIK3CA inhibitor and capivasertib is an AKT1 inhibitor.

Warnings about supplements and drug interactions

Some supplements and foods can affect the ability of a drug used to treat breast cancer to do its job. This is called a drug interaction.

You might be asked to **stop taking certain herbal supplements,** such as:

- Turmeric
- Ginkgo biloba
- Green tea extract
- St. John's Wort
- Antioxidants

Certain medicines can also affect the ability of a drug to do its job. Antacids, heart or blood pressure medicine, and antidepressants are just some of the medicines that might interact with systemic therapy or supportive care medicines given during systemic drug therapy. Therefore, it's very important to tell your care team about any medicines, vitamins, over-the-counter drugs, herbals, or supplements you're taking.

Bring a list with you to every visit.

mTOR inhibitors

mTOR is a cell protein that helps cells grow and divide. Endocrine therapy may stop working if mTOR becomes overactive. mTOR inhibitors help endocrine therapy work again.

Everolimus (Afinitor) is an mTOR inhibitor. Most often, it's taken with exemestane. For some, it may be taken with fulvestrant or tamoxifen.

Immunotherapy

Immunotherapy tries to reactivate the immune system against tumor cells. The immune system has many on and off switches. Tumors take advantage of off switches. Immunotherapy can block these off switches, which helps the immune system turn on. Immunotherapy can be given alone or with other types of treatment. Pembrolizumab and dostarlimab-gxly are immunotherapies.

Endocrine therapy

Endocrine therapy blocks estrogen or progesterone to treat hormone receptor-positive (HR+) breast cancer. The endocrine system is made up of organs and tissues that produce hormones. Hormones are natural chemicals released into the bloodstream.

There are 4 hormones that might be targeted in endocrine therapy:

- **Estrogen** is made mainly by the ovaries but is also made by other tissues in the body such as fat tissue.
- **Progesterone** is made mainly by the ovaries.
- **Luteinizing hormone-releasing hormone (LHRH)** is made by a part of the brain called the hypothalamus. It tells the ovaries to make estrogen and progesterone and testicles to make testosterone. LHRH is also called gonadotropin-releasing hormone (GnRH).
- **Androgen** is made by the adrenal glands, testicles, and ovaries.

Hormones may cause breast cancer to grow. Endocrine therapy stops your body from making hormones or blocks what hormones do in the body. This can slow cancer growth, shrink the cancer for a period of time, or prevent the cancer from returning.

Endocrine therapy is sometimes called hormone therapy or anti-estrogen therapy. It's different from hormone replacement therapy (HRT) used for menopause.

Endocrine therapy suppresses hormone production and affects the ability to become pregnant. People who want to have children in the future should be referred to a fertility specialist before starting endocrine therapy. Endocrine therapy usually lasts a minimum of 5 years but can continue up to 10 years.

Types of endocrine therapy can be found in **Guide 3**.

Testosterone

For people assigned male at birth whose bodies continue to make testosterone, endocrine therapy includes tamoxifen or an aromatase inhibitor with a testosterone-suppressing therapy.

Premenopause

If you have menstrual periods, you're in premenopause. In premenopause, the ovaries are the main source of estrogen and progesterone. People who are premenopausal must also receive ovarian ablation or suppression.

Menopause

In menopause, the ovaries permanently stop producing hormones and menstrual periods stop. Estrogen and progesterone levels are low, but the adrenal glands, liver, and body fat continue to make small amounts of estrogen. If you don't have periods, a test using a blood sample may be used to confirm your status.

Cancer treatment can cause temporary menopause. If you stopped having periods due to removal of your uterus (hysterectomy) but you still have your ovaries, then you should have your menopausal status confirmed with a blood test. If both ovaries have been removed (with or without your uterus), you're in menopause.

Preventing pregnancy during treatment

If you become pregnant during radiation therapy or endocrine therapy, it can cause birth defects. Non-hormonal birth control methods, such as intrauterine devices (IUDs) and barrier methods, are preferred in people with a breast cancer diagnosis. Types of barrier methods include condoms, diaphragms, cervical caps, and contraceptive sponges.

Guide 3
Endocrine therapy types

Bilateral oophorectomy	Surgery to remove both ovaries.
Ovarian ablation	Radiation to permanently stop the ovaries from making hormones.
Ovarian or testosterone suppression	Drugs to temporarily stop the ovaries or testicles from making hormones such as LHRH and GnRH. • LHRH agonists include Goserelin (Zoladex) and Leuprolide (Lupron Depot). These are injected every 4 or 12 weeks. They don't affect estrogen made by the ovaries. • GnRH agonists might be used to suppress ovarian hormone or testosterone production.
Aromatase inhibitors (AIs)	Drugs to stop a type of hormone called androgen from changing into estrogen by interfering with an enzyme called aromatase. AIs don't affect estrogen made by the ovaries. Nonsteroidal AIs include Anastrozole (Arimidex) and Letrozole (Femara). Exemestane (Aromasin) is a steroidal AI.
Estrogen receptor (ER) modulators or anti-estrogens	• Selective estrogen receptor modulators (SERMs) block estrogen from attaching to hormone receptors. Tamoxifen and Toremifene (Fareston) are SERMs. • Selective estrogen receptor degraders (SERDs) block and destroy estrogen receptors. Elacestrant (Orserdu), Fulvestrant (Faslodex),and Imlunestrant (Inluriyo) are SERDs.
Hormones	Examples include Estradiol, Fluoxymesterone, and Megestrol acetate (Megace).

Bone-strengthening therapy

Medicines that target the bones may be given to help relieve bone pain or reduce the risk of bone-related problems. Some medicines work by slowing or stopping bone breakdown, while others help increase bone thickness.

Inflammatory breast cancer can spread (metastasize) to your bones. This puts your bones at risk for injury and disease. Some treatments for breast cancer, like aromatase inhibitors or GnRH agonists, can cause bone loss (osteoporosis), which puts you at an increased risk for fractures.

Drugs used to prevent bone loss and fractures:

- Oral bisphosphonates
- Zoledronic acid (Zometa)
- Pamidronate (Aredia)
- Denosumab (Prolia)

Drugs used to treat bone metastases:

- Zoledronic acid (Zometa)
- Pamidronate (Aredia)
- Denosumab (Xgeva)

You may be screened for bone weakness (osteoporosis) using a bone mineral density test. This measures how much calcium and other minerals are in your bones. It's also called a dual-energy x-ray absorptiometry (DEXA) scan. Bone mineral density tests look for osteoporosis and help predict your risk for bone fractures.

Zoledronic acid, pamidronate, and denosumab

Zoledronic acid, pamidronate, and denosumab are used to prevent bone loss (osteoporosis) and fractures. Zoledronic acid and denosumab are also used in people with metastatic inflammatory breast cancer who have bone metastases to help reduce the likelihood of fractures, pain, or other complications arising from cancer in bone. You might have blood tests to monitor kidney function, calcium levels, and magnesium levels. A calcium and vitamin D supplement will likely be recommended by your doctor.

Let your dentist know if you are taking any of these medicines. Also, ask your care team how these medicines might affect your teeth and jaw. Osteonecrosis, or bone tissue death, of the jaw is a rare but serious side effect. Tell your care team about any planned trips to the dentist and surgeries or dental procedures that might also affect the jawbone. It will be important to take care of your teeth and to see a dentist before starting treatment with any of these drugs.

Clinical trials

You may also be able to receive treatment through a clinical trial. A clinical trial is a type of medical research study. After being developed and tested in a lab, potential new ways of treating cancer need to be studied in people.

If found to be safe and effective in a clinical trial, a drug, device, or treatment approach may be approved by the U.S. FDA.

Everyone with cancer should carefully consider all of the treatment options available for their cancer type, including standard treatments and clinical trials. Talk to your doctor about whether a clinical trial may make sense for you.

Phases

Most cancer clinical trials focus on treatment and are done in phases.

- **Phase 1** trials study the safety and side effects of an investigational drug or treatment approach.
- **Phase 2** trials study how well the drug or approach works against a specific type of cancer.
- **Phase 3** trials test the drug or approach against a standard treatment. If the results are good, it may be approved by the FDA.
- **Phase 4** trials study the safety and benefit of an FDA-approved treatment.

Finding a clinical trial

In the United States

NCCN Cancer Centers
NCCN.org/cancercenters

The National Cancer Institute (NCI)
cancer.gov/about-cancer/treatment/clinical-trials/search

Worldwide

The U.S. National Library of Medicine (NLM)
clinicaltrials.gov

Need help finding a clinical trial?

NCI's Cancer Information Service (CIS)
1.800.4.CANCER (1.800.422.6237)
cancer.gov/contact

Who can enroll?

It depends on the clinical trial's rules, called eligibility criteria. The rules may be about age, cancer type and stage, treatment history, or general health. They ensure that participants are alike in specific ways and that the trial is as safe as possible for the participants.

Informed consent

Clinical trials are managed by a research team. This group of experts will review the study with you in detail, including its purpose and the risks and benefits of joining. All of this information is also provided in an informed consent form. Read the form carefully and ask questions before signing it. Take time to discuss it with people you trust. Keep in mind that you can leave and seek treatment outside of the clinical trial at any time.

Will I get a placebo?

Placebos (inactive versions of real medicines) are almost never used alone in cancer clinical trials. It's common to receive either a placebo with a standard treatment, or a new drug with a standard treatment. You will be informed, verbally and in writing, if a placebo is part of a clinical trial before you enroll.

Are clinical trials free?

There's no fee to enroll in a clinical trial. The study sponsor pays for research-related costs, including the study drug. But you may need to pay for other services, like transportation or childcare, due to extra appointments. During the trial, you'll continue to receive standard cancer care. This care is often covered by insurance.

We want your feedback!

Our goal is to provide helpful and easy-to-understand information on cancer. Take our survey to let us know what we got right and what we could do better.
NCCN.org/patients/feedback

Key points

- Non-metastatic inflammatory breast cancer (IBC) is treated with systemic therapy to shrink the tumor, followed by a mastectomy, axillary lymph node dissection, and radiation therapy. Endocrine therapy will be given if the tumor is estrogen receptor-positive.
- Systemic treatment is based on estrogen receptor (ER), progesterone receptor (PR), and HER2 expression.
- Radiation therapy uses high-energy radiation from x-rays (photons, electrons), protons, and other sources to kill cancer cells.
- Some breast cancers grow because of estrogen. These cancers are estrogen receptor-positive (ER+) and are often treated with endocrine therapy to reduce the risk of cancer returning.
- Cancer can also spread to the bones. Bone-strengthening medicine helps prevent bone loss, broken bones, and bone pain.
- A clinical trial is a type of research that studies a treatment to see how safe it is and how well it works.

Questions to ask

- What is your experience treating inflammatory breast cancer?
- How many breast cancer surgeries have you done?
- What treatment will I have before and after surgery?
- How long will treatment take and in what order will it be given?
- What websites about my condition do you recommend? Is there any information I can take home to read?

What's next?

Now that you've read about the different types of treatment and what to expect, the next chapter talks about some general side effects of treatment and what might be done to manage those effects.

5

Supportive care

Supportive care helps manage the symptoms of cancer and the side effects of treatment. This chapter discusses supportive care for possible treatment side effects.

What is supportive care?

Supportive care is an important part of cancer care. The goal is to improve your quality of life during and after cancer treatment. Supportive care is for everyone with cancer and their families, not just for those at the end of life.

Supportive care includes a wide range of services. Supportive care prevents or manages the symptoms of cancer and the side effects of cancer treatment, like pain and cancer-related fatigue. It also addresses the mental, social, emotional, and spiritual concerns faced by people with cancer.

Supportive care provides help with additional needs, such as:

- Making treatment decisions
- Coordinating your care
- Paying for care
- Planning for advanced care and end of life

Read more about the types of support you may receive in *NCCN Guidelines for Patients: Palliative Care*, available at NCCN.org/patientguidelines and on the NCCN Patient Guides for Cancer app.

Side effects

All cancer treatments can cause unwanted health issues called side effects. Side effects depend on many factors. These factors include the drug type and dose, length of treatment, and the person. Some side effects may just be unpleasant. Others may be harmful to one's health. Treatment can cause several side effects. Some are very serious. Tell your care team about any new or worsening symptoms.

Some common side effects are described next.

Supportive care resources

More information on supportive care is available at NCCN.org/patientguidelines and on the NCCN Patient Guides for Cancer app.

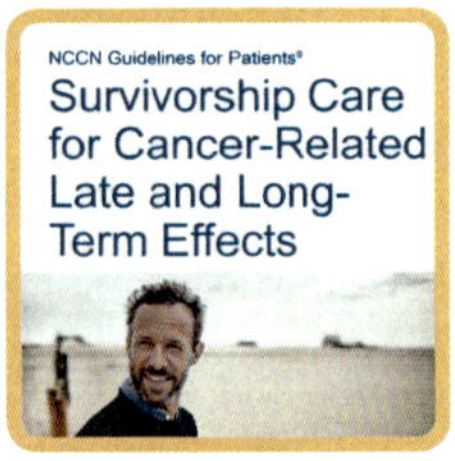

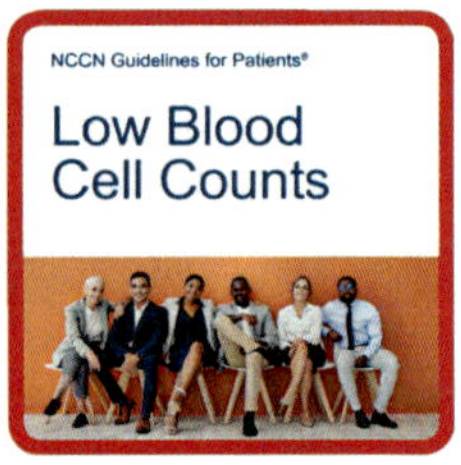

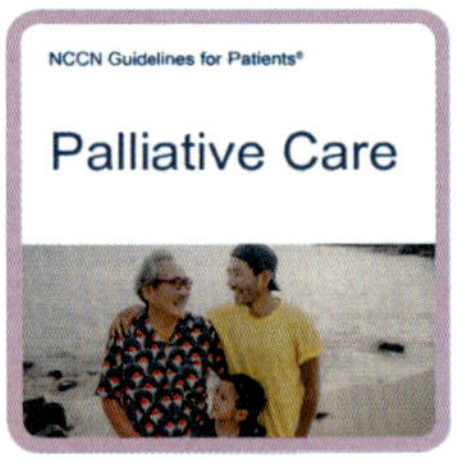

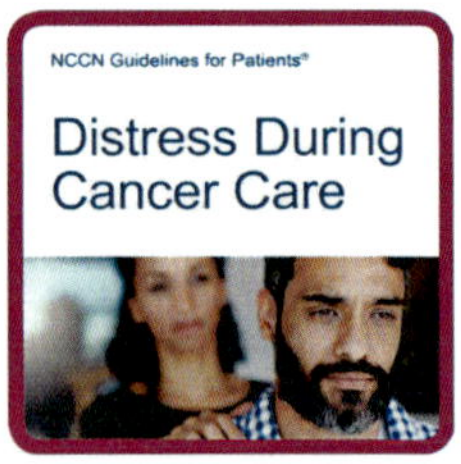

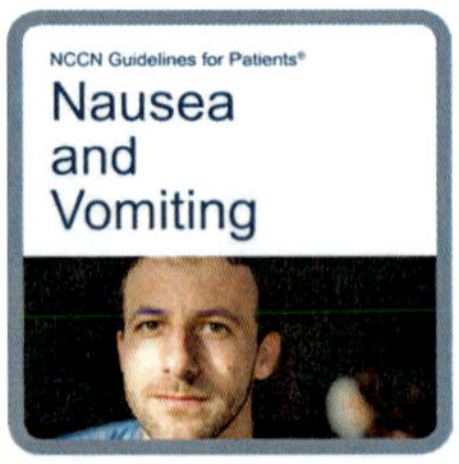

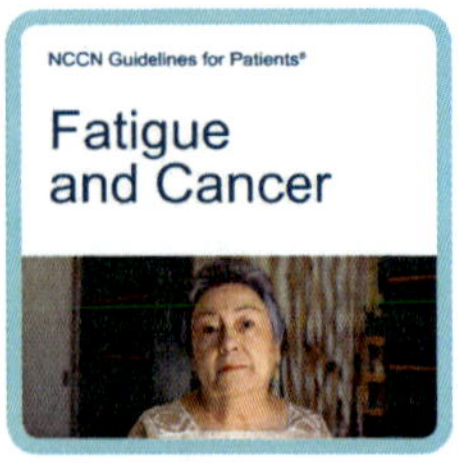

Tell your care team about all of your side effects, including new or worsening symptoms, so they can be managed.

Blood clots

Cancer treatment can cause blood clots to form. This can block blood flow and oxygen delivery to parts of the body. Blood clots can break loose and travel to other parts of the body causing breathing problems, strokes, or other problems.

Bone health

Breast cancer may spread to your bones. Some breast cancer treatments may also weaken your bones. Both can put your bones at increased risk for injury and disease. Such problems include bone fractures, bone pain, and squeezing (compression) of the spinal cord. High levels of calcium in the blood, called hypercalcemia, may also occur.

Medicine may be given to help relieve bone pain and reduce the risk of other bone problems. Some medicines work by slowing or stopping bone breakdown, while others help increase bone thickness. It's recommended that you take calcium and vitamin D with these bone health medicines. Talk to your care team first.

Diarrhea or constipation

Diarrhea is frequent and watery bowel movements. Your care team will tell you how to manage diarrhea. When it occurs, it's important to drink lots of fluids.

Constipation is also common, especially if you're taking certain pain medicines, including narcotic pain medication and some anti-nausea medications. Constipation means having less frequent and more difficult bowel movements. Drinking fluids, staying active, and taking medicines for constipation are often recommended.

Emotional distress

Depression, anxiety, and sleeping issues are common during a cancer diagnosis. Talk to your care team and those with whom you feel most comfortable about how you're feeling. There are services, people, and medicine that may be recommended to help relieve your distress.

Fatigue

Fatigue is a state of physical or mental tiredness that can feel like lack of energy, motivation, or stamina. Fatigue may be caused by cancer, or it may be a side effect of treatment. Let your care team know how you are feeling and if fatigue is getting in the way of doing the things you enjoy. Eating a balanced diet, exercise, yoga, acupuncture, and massage therapy can help. You might be referred to a nutritionist or dietitian to help with fatigue. It's important to try to stay active.

Hair loss

Chemotherapy may cause hair loss (alopecia) all over your body—not just on your scalp. Some chemotherapy drugs are more likely than others to cause hair loss. Dosage might also affect the amount of hair loss. Most of the time, hair loss from chemotherapy is temporary. Hair often regrows 3 to 6 months after treatment ends. Your hair may be a different shade or texture at first. Scalp cooling (or scalp hypothermia) might help lessen hair loss in people receiving certain types of chemotherapy.

Infections

Infections occur more frequently and are more severe in people with a weakened immune system. Drug treatment for inflammatory breast cancer can weaken the body's natural defense against infections. If not treated early, infections can be fatal.

Neutropenia, a low number of white blood cells that often occurs during treatment, can lead to frequent or severe infections. When someone with neutropenia develops a fever, it's called febrile neutropenia (FN). A fever is a temperature of over 100.4° F. With FN, your risk of infection may be higher than normal. This is because a low number of white blood cells leads to a reduced ability to fight infections. Sometimes the infection can be from bacteria entering the bloodstream, which is very dangerous. FN is a side effect of some types of systemic therapy. Ask your care team how to prevent FN, what to look for, and what to do in an emergency.

Loss of appetite

The side effects from cancer or its treatment and the stress of having cancer might cause you to feel not hungry or sick to your stomach (nauseated). You might have a sore mouth or difficulty swallowing

Healthy eating is important during treatment. It includes eating a balanced diet, eating the right amount of food, and drinking enough fluids. A registered dietitian who's an expert in nutrition and food can help.

Low blood cell counts

Some cancer treatments can cause low blood cell counts.

- **Anemia** is a condition where your body doesn't have enough healthy red blood cells, resulting in less oxygen being carried to your organs. You might tire easily if you're anemic.
- **Neutropenia** is a decrease in neutrophils, a type of white blood cell. This puts you at risk for infection.
- **Thrombocytopenia** is a condition where there aren't enough platelets found in the blood. This puts you at risk for bleeding.

Lymphedema

Lymphedema is a condition in which lymph fluid builds up in tissues and causes swelling. It may be caused when part of the lymph system is damaged or blocked, such as during surgery to remove lymph nodes, or by radiation therapy. Cancers that block lymph vessels can also cause lymphedema. Swelling usually develops slowly over time. It may develop during treatment, or it may start years after treatment. If you have lymphedema, you may be referred to an expert in lymphedema management. The swelling may be reduced by exercise, massage, compression devices, and other means.

Nausea and vomiting

Nausea and vomiting are common side effects of treatment. You may be given medicine to prevent nausea and vomiting.

Neuropathy and neurotoxicity

Some treatments can damage the nervous system (neurotoxicity) causing neuropathy and problems with concentration, memory, and thinking. Neuropathy is a nerve problem that causes pain, numbness, tingling, swelling, or muscle weakness in different parts of the body. It usually begins in the hands or feet and gets worse with additional cycles of treatment. Most of the time, neuropathy improves gradually and may eventually go away after treatment.

Pain

Tell your care team about any pain or discomfort. You might meet with a palliative care specialist or with a pain specialist to manage pain.

Late effects

Late effects are side effects that occur months or years after a disease is diagnosed or after treatment has ended. Late effects may be caused by cancer or cancer treatment. They may include physical, mental, and social health concerns, and second cancers. The sooner late effects are treated, the better. Ask your care team about what late effects could occur. This will help you know what to look for.

Survivorship

A person is a cancer survivor from the time of diagnosis until the end of life. After treatment, your health will be monitored for side effects and the return of cancer. This is part of your survivorship care plan. It's important to keep any follow-up care and imaging test appointments. Seek good routine medical care, including regular doctor visits for preventive care and cancer screening.

A personalized survivorship care plan will contain a summary of possible long-term effects of treatment called late effects and a list of follow-up tests. Find out how your primary care provider will coordinate with specialists for your follow-up care.

"It's normal to feel anxious or depressed, and there are things/medicines that can help. Make sure the people who support you also have access to this help."

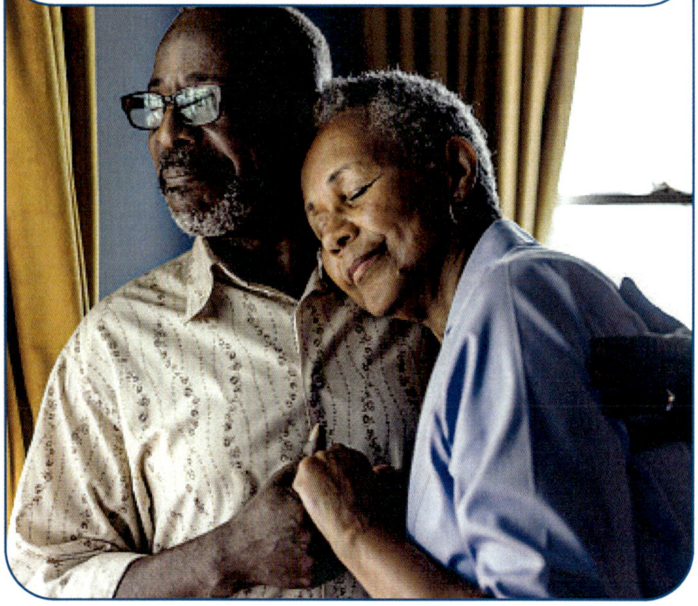

Key points

- Supportive care is health care that relieves symptoms caused by treatment and improves quality of life. Supportive care is always given.
- All cancer treatments can cause unwanted health issues called side effects. Side effects depend on many factors. These factors include the drug type and dose, length of treatment, and the person.
- Some side effects are very rare. Ask your care team what to expect.
- Tell your care team about any new or worsening symptoms.
- A person is a cancer survivor from the time of diagnosis until the end of life. After treatment, your health will be monitored for side effects of treatment and the return of cancer.

Questions to ask

- Who will coordinate my care?
- Who should I call when I have questions or notice changes in my condition?
- How long should I wait if I notice changes in my condition?
- What should I do on weekends and other non-office hours?
- Will my care team be able to communicate with the emergency department or urgent care team?

What's next?

Inflammatory breast cancer (IBC) treatment starts with drug therapy. The next chapter provides more detailed information on your treatment options before surgery.

6

Treatment before and after surgery

Since inflammatory breast cancer (IBC) spreads quickly, treatment starts with systemic (drug) therapy to stop the spread of cancer. Together, you and your care team will choose a treatment plan that's best for you.

How is inflammatory breast cancer treated?

Inflammatory breast cancer (IBC) is treated with systemic (drug) therapy to shrink the tumor, followed by surgery to remove the breast and lymph nodes (modified radical mastectomy), and then radiation therapy to the chest wall. Surgery isn't always possible. Even though surgery might not be an option, systemic therapy will continue.

If you choose breast reconstruction after a mastectomy with radiation, then delayed breast reconstruction is recommended. Radiation can slow the healing process. Therefore, it's better to wait until you have healed from radiation therapy before having breast reconstruction.

Like other breast cancers, IBC can develop in people assigned male at birth. Treatment is very similar for all genders.

Where does treatment start?

Treatment for IBC starts with preoperative systemic (drug) therapy. Preoperative therapy is treatment given before surgery. It's based on the HER2 and hormone receptor (HR) expression status of the tumor cells.

Cancer can still progress during preoperative systemic therapy. If this happens, then another systemic therapy will be given. Systemic therapy might include chemotherapy, antibody drug conjugates, or targeted therapy.

"My 3-month-old son stopped nursing on my left breast and it was swollen and painful. The doctor said it was mastitis, but this didn't feel the same as when I'd had that before. Even with the antibiotic, it didn't improve. An ultrasound showed a questionable area in that breast and a biopsy confirmed inflammatory breast cancer (IBC)."

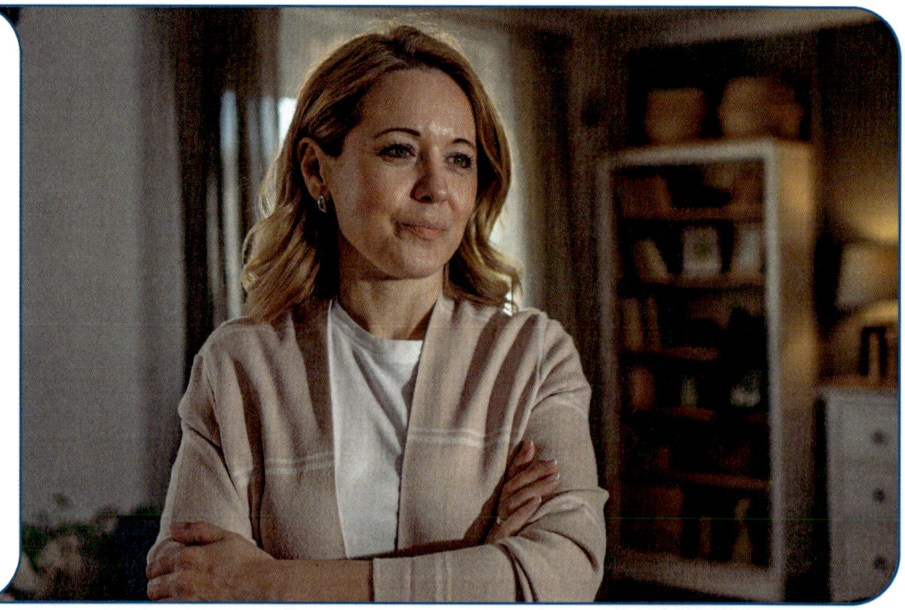

Treatment before surgery is described next.

HER2- breast cancer treatment

In HER2-negative (HER2-) breast cancer, tumor cells don't express increased levels of HER2. Chemotherapy is used to treat this type of cancer. It might include another systemic therapy. HER2- breast cancers can be hormone receptor-positive (HR+) or hormone receptor-negative (HR-).

Systemic therapy options for HER2- breast cancer can be found in **Guide 4**.

Triple-negative breast cancer

In triple-negative breast cancer (TNBC), the tumor tests negative for HER2, estrogen receptors, and progesterone receptors. It's written as ER- and/or PR- with HER2- or as HR-, HER2- This cancer is treated with chemotherapy and other systemic therapies found in **Guide 4**.

HER2+ breast cancer treatment

Inflammatory breast cancers often produce greater than normal amounts of HER2. If the tumor is HER2-positive (HER2+), then it's treated with the HER2-targeted therapy options found in **Guide 5**.

Triple-positive breast cancer

In triple-positive breast cancer, tumor cells have estrogen receptors (ER+), progesterone receptors (PR+), and a larger than normal number of HER2 receptors on their surface. It's treated with HER2-targeted therapy and endocrine therapy. A CDK4/6 inhibitor may be added. See **Guide 5**.

Treatment response

The next treatment is based on how the tumor responded to preoperative systemic therapy. It's called preoperative (before surgery) treatment because the goal is surgery, when possible. Systemic therapy given after surgery is called adjuvant therapy. Adjuvant systemic therapy may be given after surgery to reduce the chance of cancer returning, called recurrence.

A physical exam and imaging tests should be done to assess how the cancer responded to preoperative systemic therapy. Treatment is based on if the tumor can be removed with surgery or if the tumor didn't shrink enough to be removed with surgery.

Surgery is an option

If surgery is possible, then a total mastectomy with level I and II axillary lymph node dissection is recommended. Because IBC usually involves a large portion of the breast, lumpectomy isn't typically an option. You may choose a delayed breast reconstruction as part of the mastectomy. Radiation therapy is part of treatment with surgery.

Guide 4
Systemic therapy options for HER2- breast cancer

HR+, HER2- breast cancer	**Preferred therapies:** • Doxorubicin and Cyclophosphamide (AC) followed by Paclitaxel • Docetaxel and Cyclophosphamide (TC) • Olaparib, if germline *BRCA1* or *BRCA2* mutations (adjuvant only) **Other recommended therapies:** • Doxorubicin and Cyclophosphamide (AC) followed by Docetaxel • Epirubicin and Cyclophosphamide (EC) • Docetaxel, Doxorubicin, and Cyclophosphamide (TAC) **Therapies used in certain cases:** • Doxorubicin and Cyclophosphamide (AC) • Cyclophosphamide, Methotrexate, and Fluorouracil (CMF) • Doxorubicin and Cyclophosphamide (AC) followed by Paclitaxel
HR-, HER2- (triple-negative) breast cancer	**Preferred therapies:** • Preoperative Carboplatin and Paclitaxel plus Pembrolizumab, followed by preoperative Cyclophosphamide with Doxorubicin or Epirubicin plus Pembrolizumab, followed by adjuvant Pembrolizumab • If residual disease after preoperative therapy with taxane-, alkylator-, and anthracycline-based chemotherapy, then Capecitabine **Other recommended therapies:** • Drugs listed above under *HR+, HR- other recommended therapies* • Carboplatin and Paclitaxel • Carboplatin and Docetaxel **Therapies used in certain cases:** • Drugs listed above under *HR+, HR- therapies used in certain cases* • Carboplatin and Docetaxel plus Pembrolizumab (preoperative only) • Doxorubicin and Cyclophosphamide (AC) followed by Carboplatin and Docetaxel or Paclitaxel • Capecitabine (maintenance therapy after adjuvant chemotherapy)

Note: Other taxanes (ie, docetaxel, paclitaxel, albumin-bound paclitaxel) might be substituted in some cases.

Guide 5
Targeted therapy options for HER2+ breast cancer

HER2+ breast cancer	**Preferred therapies:** • Docetaxel and Carboplatin plus Trastuzumab plus Pertuzumab (TCHP) • Docetaxel and Carboplatin plus Trastuzuma (adjuvant only) If no disease remains after preoperative therapy or no preoperative therapy: • Complete up to 1 year of HER2-targeted therapy with Trastuzumab. Pertuzumab might be added. If disease remains after preoperative therapy: • Ado-trastuzumab emtansine alone. If Ado-trastuzumab emtansine discontinued for toxicity, then Trastuzumab with or without Pertuzumab to complete 1 year of therapy • If node positive at initial staging, then Trastuzumab plus Pertuzumab • Fam-trastuzumab deruxtecan-nxki (T-DXd) for those with high risk of recurrence
	Other recommended therapies: • Doxorubicin and Cyclophosphamide (AC) followed by Docetaxel plus Trastuzumab • Doxorubicin and Cyclophosphamide (AC) followed by Docetaxel plus Trastuzumab plus Pertuzumab • Carboplatin and Paclitaxel plus Pertuzumab plus Trastuzumab
	Therapies used in certain cases: • Cyclophosphamide and Docetaxel plus Trastuzumab • Doxorubicin and Cyclophosphamide (AC) followed by Paclitaxel plus Trastuzumab • Doxorubicin and Cyclophosphamide (AC) followed by Paclitaxel plus Pertuzumab plus Trastuzumab • Paclitaxel or Docetaxel plus Pertuzumab plus Trastuzumab • Neratinib (adjuvant only) • Ado-trastuzumab emtansine (TDM-1) (adjuvant only) • Paclitaxel plus Trastuzumab (adjuvant only)

Note: Other taxanes (ie, docetaxel, paclitaxel, albumin-bound paclitaxel) might be substituted in some cases.

After the mastectomy you'll finish systemic therapy if you didn't complete the course before surgery. You'll also have radiation therapy. Tumors that are estrogen receptor-positive (ER+), progesterone receptor-positive (PR+), or both (ER+/PR+) are treated with endocrine (hormone-blocking) therapy that might include CDK4/6 inhibitor therapy.

If the tumor is HER2+, then you will complete up to 1 year of HER2-targeted therapy. This may be given at the same time as radiation therapy and endocrine therapy.

- For a list of systemic therapies that target HER2+, see **Guide 5**.
- For a list of endocrine therapy options, see **Guides 6A** and **6B**.

Surgery isn't an option

Surgery isn't always possible. Even though surgery might not be an option, systemic therapy will continue. If the cancer isn't responding to systemic therapy, then radiation may be considered to try to make the cancer resectable (able to be removed with surgery). The goal of treatment is to reduce the amount of cancer. Talk with your care team about your goals of treatment and your treatment preferences. Your wishes are always important.

- For a list of systemic therapies for HER2- cancer, see **Guide 4**.
- For a list of systemic therapies that target HER2+ cancer, see **Guide 5**.

Follow-up care

After treatment, you'll receive follow-up care. During this time, your health will be monitored for side effects of treatment (late effects) and the possible return of cancer (recurrence). It's important to keep any follow-up care and imaging test appointments. Seek routine medical care, including regular doctor visits for preventive care and cancer screening. Find out who will coordinate with specialists for your follow-up care.

Tell your care team about any symptoms such as headaches, menstrual spotting between periods or new onset of spotting after menopause (if you've taken tamoxifen in the past), shortness of breath while walking, or bone pain. Side effects can be managed. Continue to take all medicine such as endocrine therapy exactly as prescribed and don't miss or skip doses.

Follow-up care can be found in **Guide 7**.

Guide 6A
Endocrine therapy for HR+ cancer – premenopausal at diagnosis

Option 1

- Tamoxifen alone or with ovarian suppression or ablation for 5 years

→

- After 5 years, if in postmenopause, then an aromatase inhibitor for 5 years or consider tamoxifen for another 5 years (for a total of 10 years on tamoxifen)
- After 5 years, if still in premenopause, then consider tamoxifen for another 5 years (for a total of 10 years on tamoxifen) or stop endocrine therapy

Option 2 (preferred for those with IBC)

- Aromatase inhibitor for 5 years with ovarian suppression or ablation, then consider aromatase inhibitor for an additional 3 to 5 years for a total of 7.5 to 10 years

Guide 6B
Endocrine therapy for HR+ cancer – menopausal at diagnosis

Option 1

- Aromatase inhibitor for 5 years, then consider aromatase inhibitor for 3 to 5 more years (for a total of 7.5 to 10 years). Preferred for those with IBC
- Aromatase inhibitor for 2 to 3 years, then tamoxifen to complete 5 years total of endocrine therapy
- Tamoxifen for 2 to 3 years, then an aromatase inhibitor to complete 5 years of endocrine therapy
- Tamoxifen for 2 to 3 years, then up to 5 years of an aromatase inhibitor

Option 2

- Tamoxifen for 4.5 to 6 years, then an aromatase inhibitor for 5 years or consider tamoxifen for another 5 years (for a total of 10 years on tamoxifen)

Option 3

- For those who can't have aromatase inhibitors or who don't want aromatase inhibitors, take tamoxifen for 5 years or consider tamoxifen for up to 10 years

Guide 7 Follow-up care
Medical history and physical exam 1 to 4 times per year as needed for 5 years, then every year
Screening for distress, anxiety, depression, and changes in family history
Genetic testing and referral to genetic counseling, as needed
Monitoring for lymphedema and refer for lymphedema management, as needed
Mammogram every 12 months (not needed for the side that underwent a mastectomy or on reconstructed breast)
Discuss issues and answer questions related to fertility, birth control, sexual health, and menopause hormone therapy (different from endocrine therapy).
Heart tests, as needed
Discuss information on risk of future health issues (comorbidities)
If signs and symptoms of metastases, then blood and imaging tests
If taking endocrine therapy, continue to take endocrine therapy. Don't miss or skip doses.
Annual gynecology exam (depending on age)
Bone density testing if you're on an aromatase inhibitor or if you have ovarian issues
Continue to see all health care providers and specialists as needed. You'll likely have to coordinate your follow-up and routine medical care appointments.
Maintain an ideal body weight (body mass index under 28), be active, eat a healthy diet, limit alcohol, and quit smoking/vaping nicotine

Key points

- Treatment for inflammatory breast cancer (IBC) starts with preoperative systemic therapy. Preoperative systemic therapy is drug treatment given before surgery. It's based on hormone receptor and HER2 expression status of the tumor cells.
- Treatment after surgery is called adjuvant treatment. It often includes systemic therapy and radiation therapy. It's given to kill any remaining cancer cells and to help prevent the return of cancer.
- Adjuvant treatment is based on cancer stage, histology, and hormone receptor status. Histology is the study of the anatomy (structure) of cells, tissues, and organs under a microscope.
- Inflammatory breast cancers often produce greater than normal amounts of HER2. If the tumor is HER2+, then HER2-targeted therapy is given.
- In hormone receptor HR-positive (HR+) cancer, tumor cells test positive for estrogen receptors, progesterone receptors, or both. Endocrine (hormone-blocking) therapy is used to treat HR+ cancer.
- If chemotherapy is given, it's given before radiation therapy and endocrine therapy.
- It's important to keep follow-up visits and imaging test appointments. Seek good routine medical care, including preventive care and cancer screenings. Continue to take all medicines as prescribed.

Questions to ask

- What treatments do you recommend and why?
- Does the order of treatments matter?
- Which option is proven to work best for my type of cancer, age, overall health, and other factors?
- Are there resources to help me pay for treatment or other care I may need?
- Am I a candidate for a clinical trial?

What's next?

The next chapter discusses how your breast might look after a mastectomy. You might consider speaking with a plastic surgeon before surgery.

Follow-up care resources

More information on follow-up care is available at NCCN.org/patientguidelines and on the NCCN Patient Guides for Cancer app.

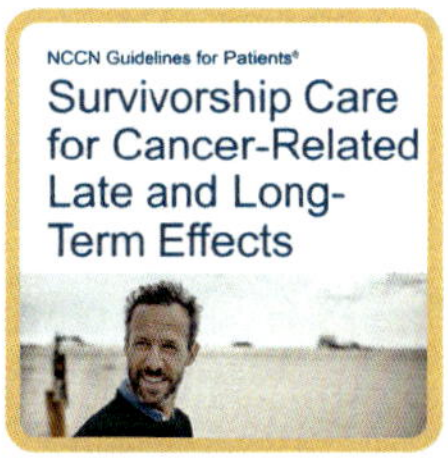

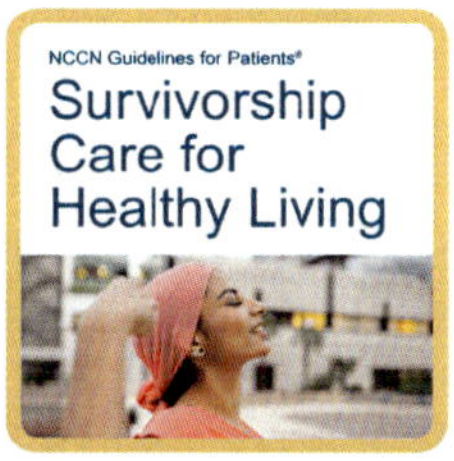

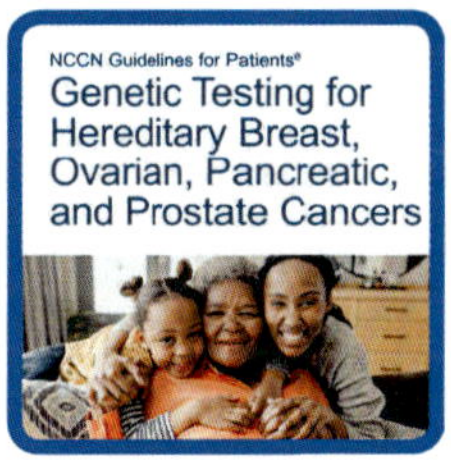

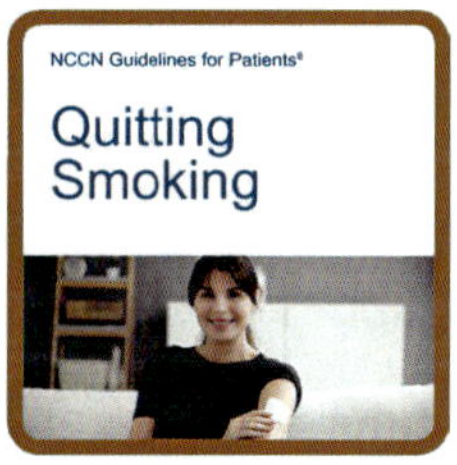

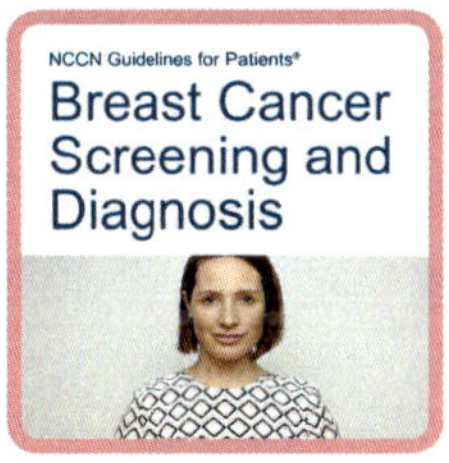

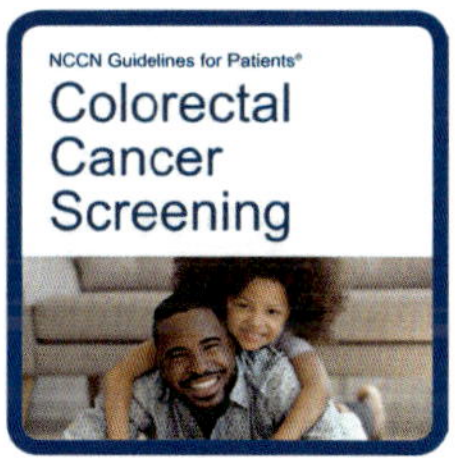

7
The breast after surgery

How your breasts look after surgery depends on the type of surgery; the amount of tissue removed; and other factors, such as your body type, age, and size and shape of the area before surgery. You might consider speaking with a plastic surgeon before surgery. This chapter offers more information on flat closure and breast reconstruction.

The recovery time for each procedure differs. This can affect your ability to return to work or participate in activities. You might consider speaking with a plastic surgeon before surgery to discuss your options and what to expect.

Flat closure after a mastectomy

In a total mastectomy with a flat closure, the entire breast, including nipple, extra skin, fat, and other tissue in the breast area, is removed. The remaining skin is tightened and sewn together. No breast mound is created, and no implant is added. The scar will be slightly raised and differ in color than the surrounding skin. A flat closure isn't completely flat or smooth. The result varies from person to person. Ask to look at pictures from flat closures so you know what to expect.

Delayed breast reconstruction after a mastectomy

Breast reconstruction is surgery to rebuild the shape and recreate the look of the breast after a mastectomy. In many cases, breast reconstruction involves a staged approach. This means it will require more than one procedure. If you opt for reconstruction, it will be done after finishing cancer treatment. This is called delayed reconstruction.

A plastic surgeon performs breast reconstruction. Breasts can be reconstructed with implants and flaps. All methods are generally safe, but as with any surgery, there are risks. Ask your treatment team for a complete list of side effects.

Implants

Breast implants are small bags filled with salt water, silicone gel, or both. They are placed under the breast skin or muscle to mimic a breast shape following a mastectomy. A balloon-like device, called an expander, may be used first to stretch out tissue. It will be placed under your skin or muscle and enlarged every few weeks for 2 to 3 months. When your skin is stretched to the proper size, you'll have surgery to place the final implant.

Implants have a small risk of leaking or causing other issues. You may feel pain from the implant or expander. Scar tissue can also arise around the implant, called capsule contracture.

Flaps

Breasts can be remade using skin from other parts of your body, known as flaps. Flaps are taken from your abdomen, buttocks, or thigh, or from under the shoulder blade. Some flaps are completely removed and then sewn in place. Other flaps stay attached to your body but are slid over and sewn into place.

There are several risks associated with flaps, including death of fat in the flap, which can cause lumps. A hernia may result from muscle weakness. Problems are more likely to occur among people who have diabetes or who smoke.

Implants and flaps

Some breasts are reconstructed with both implants and flaps. This method may give the reconstructed breast more volume to match the other breast. For any reconstruction, you may need surgery on your other breast so both breasts match.

Nipple replacement

Like your breast, a nipple can be remade. To rebuild a nipple, a plastic surgeon can use surrounding tissues, such as from the thigh or the other nipple. Tissue can be darkened with a tattoo to look more like a nipple. Also, a tattoo can be done to look like a nipple without having to take tissue from another part of the body. It's important to know that while you can remake something to look like a nipple, it won't have the sensation of your real nipple.

What to consider

Below are some factors to think about when deciding whether to have flat closure or reconstruction after mastectomy.

- **Your desire** – You may have a strong preference toward flat closure or reconstruction after being given the options. Breast reconstruction should be a shared decision between you and your care team. Make your wishes known.
- **Health issues** – You may have health issues, such as diabetes or a blood disorder, that might affect or delay healing or make longer procedures unsafe.
- **Tobacco use** – Smoking delays wound healing and can cause mastectomy flap death, nipple-areola complex death in a nipple-sparing mastectomy, infection, and failure of implant-based reconstruction. In flap reconstruction, smoking increases the risk of complications. You're encouraged to stop smoking prior to breast reconstruction surgery.
- **Breast size and shape** – There are limits to the available sizes of breast implants. Very large breasts or breasts that lack tone or droop (called ptosis) might be difficult to match. Breast reduction surgery might be an option.
- **Body mass index (BMI)** – People with a higher BMI have an increased risk of infections and complications with breast reconstruction.

Key points

- Flat closure is done after a mastectomy. The skin is tightened and sewn together without the addition of a breast implant.
- Breast reconstruction is surgery to rebuild the shape and recreate the look of the breast.
- Breasts that are fully removed in a mastectomy can be remade with breast implants, flaps, or both.
- If you opt for breast reconstruction, it will be done after completing treatment. This is called delayed breast reconstruction.
- Removed nipples can be remade with body tissue and/or tattooing.

Questions to ask

- What will my breast look like after surgery?
- How many breast surgeries or breast reconstructive surgeries have you done? What complications are possible?
- How much pain will I be in, for how long will I be in pain, and what will be done to manage my pain?
- How long does the breast reconstruction process take and what should I expect?
- What options are available if I don't like the look of my breast after surgery?

What's next?

The next chapter provides information about resources and where you can get support.

8

Other resources

Want to learn more? Here's how you can get additional help.

What else to know

This guide helps you know your options so you can make informed decisions and improve your cancer care. But it's not the only resource that you have.

Ask for as much information and help as you need. Many people are interested in learning more about:

- Finding an oncologist or surgeon who is an expert in inflammatory breast cancer
- Making treatment decisions
- The details of treatment and possible side effects
- Getting financial help
- Coping with cancer treatment and other health challenges

What else to do

Your health care center can help you with next steps. It often has on-site resources to help meet your needs and find answers to your questions. Health care centers can also inform you of resources in your community.

In addition to help from your providers, the resources listed in the next section provide support for many people like yourself.

Where to get help

Look through the list below and visit the provided websites to learn more about these organizations.

Bone Marrow & Cancer Foundation
bonemarrow.org

Breast Cancer Alliance
breastcanceralliance.org

Breastcancer.org
breastcancer.org

Brem Foundation to Defeat Breast Cancer
bremfoundation.org

CanCare, Inc.
cancare.org

Cancer*Care*
cancercare.org

Cancer Hope Network
cancerhopenetwork.org

Cancer Survivor Care
cancersurvivorcare.org

DiepC Foundation
diepcfoundation.org

FORCE: Facing Our Risk of Cancer Empowered
facingourrisk.org

GPAC Global Patient Advocacy Coalition
gpacunited.org

HIS Breast Cancer Awareness
hisbreastcancer.org

Imerman Angels
imermanangels.org

Inflammatory Breast Cancer Research Foundation
ibcresearch.org

Lobular Breast Cancer Alliance
lobularbreastcancer.org

PAN Foundation
panfoundation.org

Sharsheret
sharsheret.org

Stupid Cancer
stupidcancer.org

Triage Cancer
triagecancer.org

Unite for HER
uniteforher.org

Young Survival Coalition (YSC)
youngsurvival.org

Questions to ask

- Who can I talk to about help with housing, food, and other basic needs?
- What help is available for transportation, childcare, and home care?
- What other services are available to me and my caregivers?
- How can I connect with others and build a support system?
- Who can I talk to if I don't feel safe at home, at work, or in my neighborhood?

"Be your own advocate. Talk to someone who has gone through the same thing as you. Ask a lot of questions, even the ones you are afraid to ask. You have to protect yourself and ensure you make the best decisions for you, and get the best care for your particular situation."

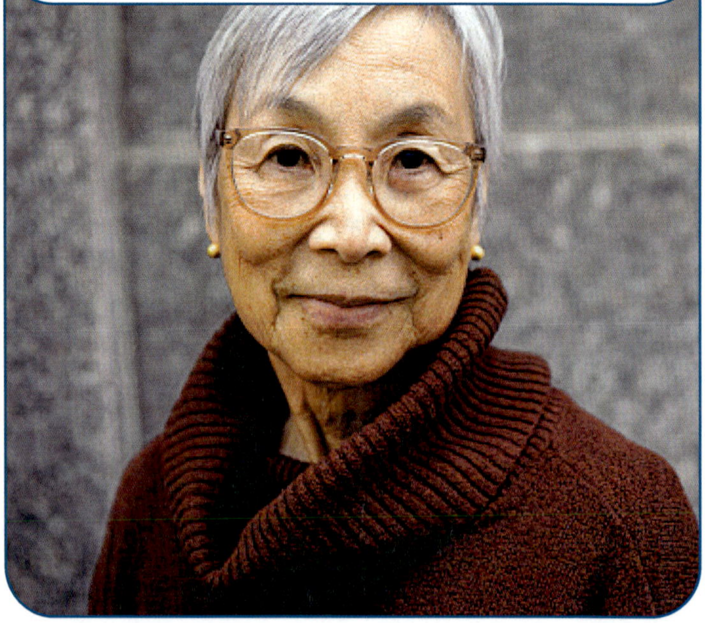

Words to know

antibody drug conjugate (ADC)
A substance made of a protein linked to a drug that attaches and enters certain types of cancer cells.

anti-estrogen
A drug that stops estrogen from attaching to cells.

areola
A darker, round area of skin on the breast around the nipple.

aromatase inhibitor (AI)
A drug that lowers estrogen levels.

axillary lymph node (ALN)
A small, disease-fighting structure near the armpit (axilla).

axillary lymph node dissection (ALND)
An operation that removes lymph nodes near the armpit.

bilateral oophorectomy
An operation that removes both ovaries.

biopsy
A procedure that removes fluid or tissue samples to be tested for a disease.

bone mineral density
A test that measures the strength of bones.

bone scan
A test that makes pictures of bones to look for health problems.

breast implant
A small bag filled with salt water, gel, or both used to remake breasts.

breast reconstruction
An operation that creates new breasts.

cancer stage
A rating of the outlook of a cancer based on its growth and spread.

chest wall
The layer of muscle, bone, and fat that protects the vital organs.

clinical breast exam
Touching of a breast by a health expert to feel for diseases.

clinical stage (c)
The rating of the extent of cancer before treatment is started.

clinical trial
A type of research that assesses health tests or treatments.

contrast
A substance put into your body to make clearer pictures during imaging tests.

core needle biopsy
A procedure that removes tissue samples with a hollow needle. Also called core biopsy.

diagnostic mammogram
Pictures made from x-rays that are focused on specific areas inside of the breasts.

duct
A tube-shaped structure through which milk travels to the nipple.

endocrine therapy
A cancer treatment that stops the making or action of estrogen. Also called hormone therapy.

estrogen
A hormone that plays a role in breast development.

estrogen receptor (ER)
A protein inside cells that binds to estrogen.

estrogen receptor-negative (ER-)
A type of breast cancer that doesn't use estrogen to grow.

estrogen receptor-positive (ER+)
A type of breast cancer that uses estrogen to grow.

fertility specialist
An expert who helps people have babies.

fine-needle aspiration (FNA)
A procedure that removes tissue samples with a very thin needle.

flat closure
A procedure done after a mastectomy in which the skin is tightened and sewn together without the addition of a breast implant.

gene
Coded instructions in cells for making new cells and controlling how cells behave.

genetic counseling
Expert guidance on the chance for a disease passed down in families.

hereditary breast cancer
Breast cancer likely caused by abnormal genes passed down from biological parent to child.

histology
The structure of cells, tissues, and organs as viewed under a microscope.

hormone
A chemical that triggers a response from cells or organs.

hormone receptor-negative cancer (HR-)
Cancer cells that don't use hormones to grow.

hormone receptor-positive cancer (HR+)
Cancer cells that use hormones to grow.

human epidermal growth factor receptor 2 (HER2)
A protein on the surface of a cell that sends signals for the cell to grow.

immunohistochemistry (IHC)
A lab test of cancer cells to find specific cell traits involved in abnormal cell growth.

inflammatory breast cancer (IBC)
A type of breast cancer in which the breast looks red and swollen and feels warm to the touch.

infraclavicular
The area right below the collarbone.

in situ hybridization (ISH)
A lab test that counts the number of copies of a gene.

internal mammary
The area along the breastbone.

invasive breast cancer
The growth of breast cancer into the breast's supporting tissue.

lobule
A gland in the breast that makes breast milk.

luteinizing hormone-releasing hormone (LHRH)
A hormone in the brain that helps control the making of estrogen by the ovaries.

lymph
A clear fluid containing white blood cells.

lymphedema
Swelling caused by a buildup of fluid called lymph.

lymph node
A small, bean-shaped, disease-fighting structure.

magnetic resonance imaging (MRI)
A test that uses radio waves and powerful magnets to take pictures of the inside of the body.

mammogram
A picture of the inside of the breast made using x-rays.

mastectomy
An operation that removes the whole breast.

menopause
12 months after the last menstrual period.

modified radical mastectomy
An operation that removes the whole breast and lymph nodes under the arm (axilla).

mutation
An abnormal change.

nipple-areola complex (NAC)
The ring of darker breast skin is called the areola. The raised tip within the areola is called the nipple.

pathologic stage (p)
A rating of the extent of cancer given after examining tissue removed during surgery.

pathologist
A doctor who's an expert in testing cells and tissue to find disease.

positron emission tomography (PET)
A test that uses radioactive material to see the shape and function of body parts.

premenopause
The state of having menstrual periods.

progesterone (PR)
A hormone involved in sexual development, menstrual periods, and pregnancy.

prognosis
The likely course and outcome of a disease based on tests.

radiation therapy (RT)
A treatment that uses high-energy rays. Also called radiotherapy.

radical mastectomy
An operation that removes the whole breast, lymph nodes under the arm (axilla), and chest wall muscles under the breast.

recurrence
The return of cancer after a cancer-free period.

selective estrogen receptor degrader (SERD)
A drug that blocks and destroys estrogen receptors.

selective estrogen receptor modulator (SERM)
A drug that blocks the effect of estrogen inside of cells.

side effect
An unhealthy or unpleasant physical or emotional response to treatment.

supportive care
Health care that includes symptom relief but not cancer treatment. Also called palliative care or best supportive care.

supraclavicular
The area right above the collarbone.

systemic therapy
Drug treatment that works throughout the body.

TNM score
A system used to stage breast cancer. The letters T (tumor), N (node), and M (metastasis) describe different areas of cancer growth.

total mastectomy
An operation that removes the entire breast with a flat closure. Also called simple mastectomy.

triple-negative breast cancer (TNBC)
Breast cancer that doesn't use hormones or the HER2 protein to grow.

NCCN Contributors

This patient guide is based on the NCCN Clinical Practice Guidelines in Oncology (NCCN Guidelines®) for Breast Cancer, Version 2.2026. It was adapted, reviewed, and published with help from the following people:

Dorothy A. Shead, MS
Senior Director
Patient Information Operations

Tanya Fischer, MEd, MSLIS
Senior Medical Writer

Lisa Diehl
Production Layout Artist

The NCCN Clinical Practice Guidelines in Oncology (NCCN Guidelines®) for Breast Cancer, Version 2.2026, were developed by the following NCCN Panel Members:

*William J. Gradishar, MD/Chair
Robert H. Lurie Comprehensive Cancer Center of Northwestern University

Meena S. Moran, MD/Vice-Chair
Yale Cancer Center/Smilow Cancer Hospital

Jame Abraham, MD
Case Comprehensive Cancer Center/ University Hospitals Seidman Cancer Center and Cleveland Clinic Taussig Cancer Institute

Vandana Abramson, MD
Vanderbilt-Ingram Cancer Center

Rebecca Aft, MD, PhD
Siteman Cancer Center at Barnes-Jewish Hospital and Washington University School of Medicine

Doreen Agnese, MD
The Ohio State University Comprehensive Cancer Center - James Cancer Hospital and Solove Research Institute

Kimberly H. Allison, MD
Stanford Cancer Institute

*Bethany Anderson, MD
University of Wisconsin Carbone Cancer Center

Janet Bailey, MD
University of Michigan Rogel Cancer Center

Harold J. Burstein, MD, PhD
Dana-Farber/Brigham and Women's Cancer Center

Nan Chen, MD
The UChicago Medicine Comprehensive Cancer Center

Helen Chew, MD
UC Davis Comprehensive Cancer Center

Chau Dang, MD
Memorial Sloan Kettering Cancer Center

Anthony D. Elias, MD
University of Colorado Cancer Center

Sharon H. Giordano, MD, MPH
The University of Texas MD Anderson Cancer Center

Matthew P. Goetz, MD
Mayo Clinic Comprehensive Cancer Center

Rachel C. Jankowitz, MD
Abramson Cancer Center at the University of Pennsylvania

Sara H. Javid, MD
Fred Hutchinson Cancer Center

A. Marilyn Leitch, MD
UT Southwestern Simmons Comprehensive Cancer Center

Janice Lyons, MD
Case Comprehensive Cancer Center/ University Hospitals Seidman Cancer Center and Cleveland Clinic Taussig Cancer Institute

Susie McCloskey, MD, MSHS
UCLA Jonsson Comprehensive Cancer Center

Melissa McShane, MD
Fox Chase Cancer Center

Sameer A. Patel, MD
Fox Chase Cancer Center

Laura H. Rosenberger, MD, MS
Duke Cancer Institute

Hope S. Rugo, MD
UCSF Helen Diller Family Comprehensive Cancer Center

Cesar A. Santa-Maria, MD, MSCI
Johns Hopkins Kimmel Cancer Center

Bryan P. Schneider, MD
Indiana University Melvin and Bren Simon Comprehensive Cancer Center

Mary Lou Smith, JD, MBA
Research Advocacy Network

Hatem Soliman, MD
Moffitt Cancer Center

*Corey Speers, MD, PhD
O'Neal Comprehensive Cancer Center at UAB

Melinda L. Telli, MD
Stanford Cancer Institute

*Mei Wei, MD
Huntsman Cancer Institute at the University of Utah

Kari B. Wisinski, MD
University of Wisconsin Carbone Cancer Center

Amulya Yellala, MBBS
Fred & Pamela Buffett Cancer Center

Kay T. Yeung, MD, PhD
UC San Diego Moores Cancer Center

Jessica S. Young, MD
Roswell Park Comprehensive Cancer Center

NCCN

Rashmi Kumar, PhD
Senior Director, Clinical Content

Ryan Schonfeld, BA
Manager, Guidelines Development Processes

* Reviewed this patient guide. For disclosures, visit NCCN.org/disclosures.

NCCN Cancer Centers

For contact information, visit NCCN.org/cancercenters.

Abramson Cancer Center
at the University of Pennsylvania
Philadelphia, Pennsylvania

Case Comprehensive Cancer Center/
University Hospitals Seidman Cancer Center and
Cleveland Clinic Taussig Cancer Institute
Cleveland, Ohio

City of Hope National Medical Center
Duarte, California

Dana-Farber Cancer Institute
Boston, Massachusetts

Duke Cancer Institute
Durham, North Carolina

Fox Chase Cancer Center
Philadelphia, Pennsylvania

Fred & Pamela Buffett Cancer Center
Omaha, Nebraska

Fred Hutchinson Cancer Center
Seattle, Washington

Huntsman Cancer Institute at the University of Utah
Salt Lake City, Utah

Indiana University Melvin and Bren Simon
Comprehensive Cancer Center
Indianapolis, Indiana

Johns Hopkins Kimmel Cancer Center
Baltimore, Maryland

Mass General Brigham Cancer Institute
Boston, Massachusetts

Mayo Clinic Comprehensive Cancer Center
Phoenix/Scottsdale, Arizona
Jacksonville, Florida
Rochester, Minnesota

Memorial Sloan Kettering Cancer Center
New York, New York

Moffitt Cancer Center
Tampa, Florida

O'Neal Comprehensive Cancer Center at UAB
Birmingham, Alabama

Robert H. Lurie Comprehensive Cancer Center
of Northwestern University
Chicago, Illinois

Roswell Park Comprehensive Cancer Center
Buffalo, New York

Siteman Cancer Center at Barnes-Jewish Hospital
and WashU Medicine
St. Louis, Missouri

St. Jude Children's Research Hospital/
The University of Tennessee Health Science Center
Memphis, Tennessee

Stanford Cancer Institute
Stanford, California

The Ohio State University Comprehensive Cancer Center -
James Cancer Hospital and Solove Research Institute
Columbus, Ohio

The UChicago Medicine Comprehensive Cancer Center
Chicago, Illinois

The University of Texas MD Anderson Cancer Center
Houston, Texas

UC Davis Comprehensive Cancer Center
Sacramento, California

UC San Diego Moores Cancer Center
La Jolla, California

UCLA Jonsson Comprehensive Cancer Center
Los Angeles, California

UCSF Helen Diller Family Comprehensive Cancer Center
San Francisco, California

University of Colorado Cancer Center
Aurora, Colorado

University of Michigan Rogel Cancer Center
Ann Arbor, Michigan

University of Wisconsin Carbone Cancer Center
Madison, Wisconsin

UT Southwestern Simmons
Comprehensive Cancer Center
Dallas, Texas

Vanderbilt-Ingram Cancer Center
Nashville, Tennessee

Yale Cancer Center/Smilow Cancer Hospital
New Haven, Connecticut

Index